COLLAGEN

Self-Care Secrets to Eat, Drink, and Glow

Jessica Bippen, MS, RD

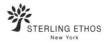

STERLING ETHOS
New York

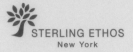

STERLING ETHOS
New York

An Imprint of Sterling Publishing Co., Inc.
1166 Avenue of the Americas
New York. NY 10036

ISBN 978-1-4549-3780-7

Distributed in Canada by Sterling Publishing Co., Inc.
c/o Canadian Manda Group, 664 Annette Street
Toronto, Ontario M6S 2C8, Canada
Distributed in the United Kingdom by GMC Distribution Services
Castle Place, 166 High Street, Lewes, East Sussex BN7 1XU, England
Distributed in Australia by NewSouth Books
University of New South Wales, Sydney, NSW 2052, Australia

For information about custom editions, special sales, and premium
and corporate purchases, please contact Sterling Special Sales at
800-805-5489 or specialsales@sterlingpublishing.com.

Manufactured in Canada

2 4 6 8 10 9 7 5 3 1

sterlingpublishing.com

Cover design by David Ter-Avanesyan
Photographs by: Jessica Bippen
Collagen Triple Helix: Shutterstock/StudioMolekuul 5,
Icons: Brickclay/Getty Images (throughout)

CONTENTS

INTRODUCTION

Collagen is showing up everywhere. What used to be touted by the beauty industry as a miracle worker for a youthful appearance is now taking over the health and wellness world. You can find it in coffee creamers, nut butter, protein bars, and even water. It's easy to find collagen supplements in the form of powders, capsules, and gummies. But what exactly is collagen and why is it so popular?

Collagen is a protein found in all animals. In humans, collagen makes up one-third of all the protein content in the body and is the main component of its various connective tissues. The beauty and wellness world has begun promoting ingestible collagen supplements as a means to help boost the body's natural levels of collagen. Collagen helps give strength and structure to our bones, muscles, skin, and tendons. It also helps to reduce the seemingly inevitable signs of aging, including saggy skin, wrinkles, and weaker joints. Using supplemental collagen for these purposes may seem far-fetched, but these products mimic the ancient practice of consuming collagen-rich bone broths made from animal bones and tissues to support youthful skin and bones.

Many cultures around the world take part in "nose-to-tail eating." Simmering bones, along with the tendons and flesh of fish, chicken, and other animals into broths that are used as bases for soups and stews, makes sure no parts of the animal go to waste. This zero-waste way of incorporating collagen-rich parts of animals dates back to the Paleolithic period and has been noted in records in many places around the globe. In fact, this way of eating is still very much a part of many cuisines.

Those living in Western countries often don't consume collagen-rich foods on a daily basis and may even find them unappetizing. Health-conscious consumers are removing the skin from poultry and fish and choosing lean cuts of meat to reduce their intake of saturated fats.

Many people are reducing their meat and animal protein consumption altogether for health and environmental reasons.

It wasn't until recently that it became possible to isolate collagen for consumption in the form of supplements. This approach has allowed people to benefit from collagen without having to consume its whole-food forms. With more research backing up the claims about the benefits of collagen, more dietitians, nutritionists, and medical practitioners recommend incorporating it into your daily diet.

As a dietitian, I love science. I like to understand why a particular food is beneficial and how it works in the body. As soon as collagen started attracting attention in the wellness world, I approached it with curiosity and skepticism. Digging into the research showed me that collagen offered benefits and why it was gaining in popularity.

The next step was to try it for myself. I began mixing collagen peptides into my coffee, tea, smoothies, yogurt, and peanut butter. You name it, I've probably mixed collagen powder into it! After about three months of taking about 20 grams of collagen peptides daily, I found my hair was growing rapidly and appeared thicker. My nails grew quickly as well. I noticed fewer of those little fine lines around my mouth and eyes. My skin felt plumper and tauter and stayed hydrated throughout the winter.

Consider this book your ultimate guide to collagen. It offers a simple but science-based look into collagen and its benefits and will help you decide whether collagen supplements are right for you. You'll find thirty-three delicious, healthy recipes that showcase how to incorporate a daily dose of collagen while maintaining a plant-centered diet.

Before you dive in, I want to remind you that studies on the effects of collagen are new. As with most things in nutrition, there is a lot we still don't know. I encourage you to keep an open mind. You are a unique individual, and even if new science deems the results of ingesting collagen inconclusive, you may just find that taking it works wonders!

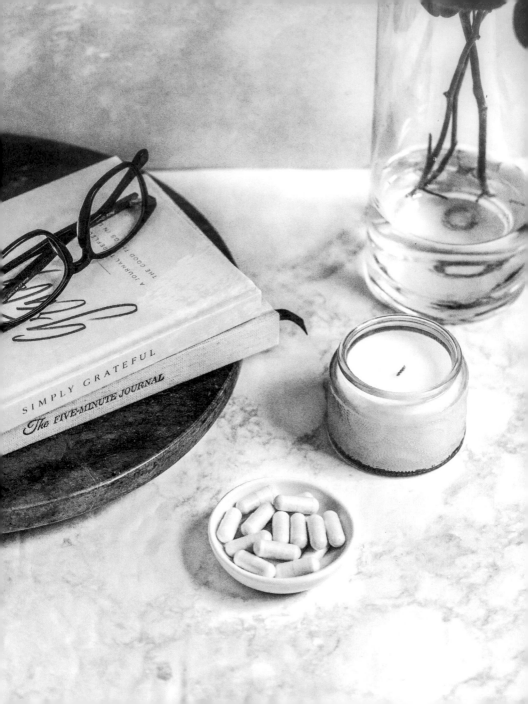

· CHAPTER ONE ·

WHAT IS COLLAGEN?

Collagen is a unique protein found in all animals. Think of collagen as the "glue" that holds your body together. It supports our bones, blood vessels, skin, cartilage, tendons, hair, nails, joints, and even our guts. Needless to say, it's a pretty important part of the body!

To fully understand how collagen forms, its functions in the body, and its benefits, let's take a closer look at the science behind this protein.

PROTEIN AND AMINO ACIDS

Protein is one of the three macronutrients—carbohydrates, fat, and protein—that are the main components of the food you eat. It's made from twenty amino acids that bind together in different ways to create the different types of protein found throughout the body.

Our amazing bodies can make eleven of the twenty amino acids, but we need to get the other nine through our diet. These nine amino acids are categorized as essential amino acids. The other eleven are considered nonessential because we can make them "in-house."

There are several nonessential amino acids that are classified as conditionally essential, meaning they become essential under specific circumstances, such as infancy, illness, or stress. During these times, the body's demand for these nonessential amino acids exceeds the amount that the body can produce. To meet this high demand, you must get these conditionally essential amino acids from your diet. For example, cystine is considered a conditionally essential amino acid in times of stress, because it is required to synthesize glutathione, an antioxidant that plays a key role during tissue repair and collagen synthesis and can be depleted by physical and emotional stressors. Arginine, glutamine, and cystine also become conditionally essential amino acids when your body needs to heal wounds. Whether you need a boost of nonessential amino acids from your diet will depend on your overall health and stress levels.

Essential Amino Acids

- histidine
- isoleucine
- leucine
- lysine
- methionine
- phenylalanine
- threonine
- tryptophan
- valine

Nonessential Amino Acids

- alanine
- arginine
- asparagine
- aspartic acid
- cysteine
- glutamic acid
- glutamine
- glycine
- proline
- serine
- tyrosine

Conditional Amino Acids

- arginine
- cysteine
- glutamine
- glycine
- proline
- serine
- tyrosine

When you consume protein, it gets broken down into amino acids in the digestive tract and contributes to the body's pool of amino acids Since different forms of protein are made up of different amino acid combinations, the types of amino acids in the pool will vary depending on what you eat.

Your body dips into this pool, combining amino acids into various structures to form all the different proteins that it needs. Since our bodies are working around the clock to constantly repair, rebuild, and function optimally, we need a constant supply of amino acids. This is why it's so important to make sure we are eating enough protein each day and are eating it throughout the day. We need to make sure we are constantly maintaining the supply of our amino acid pool—especially those essential amino acids we can get only through our diet.

THE STRUCTURE OF COLLAGEN

Collagen contains eighteen of the twenty amino acids found in the human body, including eight out of the nine essential amino acids. Since collagen does not contain tryptophan, one of the essential amino acids, it's considered an incomplete protein.

Collagen is a fibrous protein that tends to be somewhat linear in shape. Like other proteins, collagen begins with amino acids as its building blocks. The amino acids that form collagen come together to form three polypeptide chains, which are chains consisting of two or three amino acids. Most of these chains are made up of glycine, proline, hydroxylysine, and hydroxyproline. Of these amino acids, hydroxylysine and hydroxyproline are the ones not found in other proteins in our bodies. These polypeptide chains are cross-linked for strength and form into a helical arrangement, making a tough, rod-like structure known as a triple helix.

Collagen polypeptides can also be attached to carbohydrate chains, making them glycoproteins. Glycoproteins are needed in nearly every process that takes place inside our cells. They have a large role

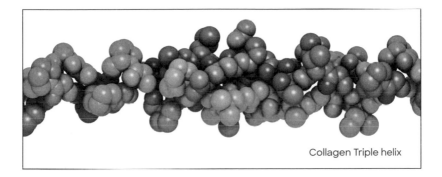

Collagen Triple helix

in supporting our immune system, digestive system, hormones, and reproductive system.

Types of Collagen

There are twenty-eight different types of collagen found in the various structural tissues throughout the body. These twenty-eight types of collagen are categorized into five main types, with most of the collagen in your body consisting of types I, II, and III.

Each type of collagen has a unique amino acid makeup and physical structure, which determines the specific role and function of that type of collagen in the body. For instance, joint cartilage has a different amino acid combination and structure than the collagen found in the lining of the gut. Types I, II, and III all have the same structure: a triple helix. This means that the strands of amino acids are wound together to create an incredibly strong, coiled molecule. Gram for gram, type I collagen is stronger than steel.

Type I is by far the most common form of collagen in the body, followed by type III. These two types of collagen make up the components of the skin, bones, tendons, and connective tissues. However, each of the five main types of collagen plays an important role in many of the structural components in the body.

TYPE I: This is the most abundant type of collagen, making up about 90 percent of the collagen in your body. It's found in almost every tissue, including the skin, bones, teeth, tendons, cartilage, and connective tissues. It's made up of densely packed fibers, which give these structures their incredible strength and elasticity. As type I collagen degrades, it's most apparent in the skin. You'll begin to notice wrinkles, saggy skin, and loss of elasticity in the skin. Type I collagen is also present in scar tissue. Cells surrounding wounded tissues create these densely packed fibers as a repair mechanism.

TYPE II: This type of collagen is made of more loosely packed fibers. It's the collagen primarily found in cartilage, which provides the cushion and padding for the end of our long bones and joints. Cartilage protects these bones from grinding together. Type II collagen is found in other places throughout the body, including the cartilage in the ear, nose, bronchial tubes, and rib cage.

TYPE III: The majority of type III collagen is found alongside type I collagen. It is also the main component of reticular fibers. Reticular fibers act as a supporting mesh in soft tissues, such as the liver, bone marrow, and the tissues and organs of the lymphatic system. Type III collagen helps support the structure of muscles, blood vessels, and internal organs, including the uterus.

TYPE IV: This type of collagen doesn't form a fibrous triple-helix structure like types I, II, and III collagen. Instead, it creates a weblike pattern. Type IV collagen is unique to the basal lamina, also known as the basement membrane. The basement membrane makes up a thin layer outside the cells, giving the outer cell layer structure and helping with filtration through the cells. It's also found in the skin, liver, kidneys, and other internal organs.

TYPE V: Type V collagen helps form cell surfaces and hair. It's also required to form the cells that create a pregnant woman's placenta. The placenta is the essential organ that develops inside the uterus and attaches to the uterine wall during pregnancy. It provides a constant supply of oxygen and nutrients to the baby and removes waste products from the baby's blood.

If you're feeling overwhelmed, don't worry! Knowing the types of collagen is helpful for understanding what collagen is on a biological level, but don't let this information trip you up if you're looking to purchase collagen supplements. Your body breaks down all proteins, including collagen, into their various amino acids or polypeptides. Although it's true that there are twenty-eight types of collagen, the specific type you consume isn't going to make a difference. You may see things like "Type I and III" or "Type II" on a collagen supplement label. This can tell you a little bit about what part of the animal the collagen comes from, but more than anything it's a marketing ploy. If you consume types I and III collagen, it doesn't automatically rebuild the type I and type III collagen in your body.

Right now, there is no recommendation that humans should consume one type of collagen over another. When it comes down to it, collagen is collagen. Even though the amino acid combination for each type of collagen differs slightly, the types of collagen proteins found in the various tissues are always the same regardless of the source. The collagen proteins making up tendons in cows are no different from the collagen found in human tendons. And all types of collagen can benefit your hair, skin, nails, bones, and joints.

COLLAGEN PRODUCTION IN THE BODY

Our bodies make collagen using the amino acids from the protein we eat, along with key vitamins and minerals needed for collagen production. When we have enough of the amino acids and other nutrients needed for collagen production, we can rebuild collagen throughout the body. The exact amino acid composition for each type of collagen varies depending on the type of tissue being made and the method of preparation inside our cells.

It is essential that we consume the necessary amount of protein daily to maintain our amino acids pool and produce collagen. Our outward appearance, along with the integrity of our organs, tendons, and blood vessels, depends on our body's collagen production. The Recommended Dietary Allowance (RDA) for protein is 0.8 grams of protein per kilogram of body weight, or 0.36 grams per pound. Collagen production also needs assistance from numerous vitamins, minerals, and other nutrients to form high-quality structures. Vitamin C, copper, iron, zinc, and silicon all play a role in the intricate formation of the various collagen proteins. These will be discussed in more detail a little later in the book (see pages 20–25), so hang tight!

What Causes Loss of Collagen?

The body has the incredible ability to create collagen. Unfortunately, collagen loss is inevitable and an unavoidable part of the aging process, and there are multiple factors that can accelerate the rate of collagen breakdown. Ten top collagen killers are covered here.

Age

As we age, the collagen in our bodies begins to deteriorate, and our natural collagen production slows. This process starts when we are about 25 years old, collagen production decreases at a rate of 1 percent each year and at a higher rate in women after menopause. Studies show that even in sun-protected skin, collagen production decreases by approximately 75 percent in those older than eighty compared with those between ages eighteen and twenty-nine. Old skin has 60 percent less collagen than young skin.

As collagen production starts to decline, the seemingly inevitable signs of aging, including saggy skin, wrinkles, more pronounced cellulite, weaker joints, brittle hair and nails, and digestion issues begin to show up. The "glue" that holds your body together, providing strength and structure to your tissues, is now breaking down. Instead of reveling in taut, glowing, youthful-looking skin and a strong, flexible body, you start to notice the classic signs of aging. This breakdown of collagen can also lead to joint pain, digestive issues, and bone loss, to name just a few problems. Prevention is key to minimizing the effects of aging. Adopting a healthy diet and lifestyle practices that reduce the acceleration of collagen loss are essential for aging gracefully. This includes eating a well-balanced diet with minimal sugar and few heavily processed foods, managing stress levels, getting adequate sleep, and wearing sunscreen.

Diet

A diet full of ultra-processed foods, refined sugar and carbohydrates, and inflammatory oils that are high in omega-6 fatty acids is a top collagen killer. These foods spike blood sugar, which increases the rate of glycation—a process in which blood sugars attach to proteins to form new molecules called advanced glycation end products (AGEs). AGEs damage nearby proteins and can make collagen dry, brittle, and weak.

Cookies, chips, and baked goods are common examples of ultra-processed and high-sugar foods, but don't forget to watch out for packaged foods that have unnecessary added sugars, such as store-bought nut butters, condiments, and sauces, and inflammatory oils including soybean oil and canola oil.

Instead of choosing these ultra-processed, inflammatory foods, nourish your body with nutrient-dense whole foods. You can satisfy your sweet tooth with natural sugars found in fruits and vegetables, such as berries, watermelon, oranges, carrots, and sweet potatoes. Choose whole-food sources of carbohydrates, such as whole grains, jasmine or basmati rice, sweet potatoes, and other starchy vegetables like butternut squash, pumpkin, and other winter squashes. Avoid inflammatory oils by reading labels and opt for healthy oils like olive oil, avocado oil, and ghee, or fats from such whole foods as nuts, seeds, avocados, and coconut.

Sunlight

Sun exposure is one of the biggest contributors to accelerated collagen breakdown and cellular aging. Ultraviolet rays from the sunlight cause collagen to break down more rapidly by damaging collagen fibers and causing abnormal elastin to build up. Elastin is another type of protein found in the skin that helps provide structure. When the connective tissues such as collagen and elastin rebuild incorrectly, wrinkles form.

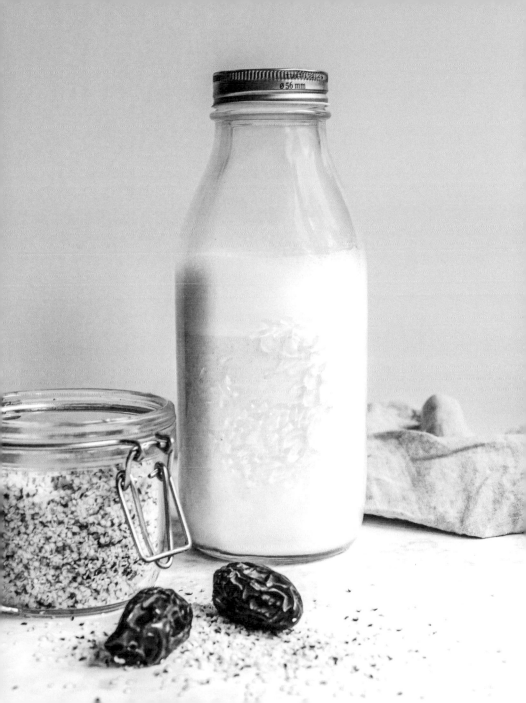

One of the easiest ways to protect your skin is to use nontoxic, mineral-based sunscreen that protects against both UVA and UVB rays. Look for a sunscreen with an SPF of at least 35.

Stress

Have you ever noticed that a president seems to age by twenty years after completing a term in office? Or maybe you've had a friend or family member go through a loss or illness that's suddenly caused them to look much older. The common factor here is stress. Stress makes our cells age at a rapid pace.

The body experiences stress when a person feels the effects of mental, physical, or emotional pressure. When the body perceives stress, the body releases cortisol, its primary stress hormone. Constant stress causes the body to increase its production of cortisol, which contributes to increased inflammation and disrupts proper cellular function, including the production of collagen and elastin. This is most noticeable in the skin, appearing as sagginess and wrinkles.

To cope with stress, incorporate a stress-management practice like meditation, journaling, spending time in nature, positive affirmations and self-talk, or therapy. I also recommend adding restorative movement and low-impact exercise, such as walking or yoga, to your daily routine, along with B vitamins. Stress depletes the body's level of B vitamins, which are essential for calming down your nervous system.

Sleep

Sleep is vital for your overall health. It's when your body, including your skin, repairs itself. When sleep is compromised, the body's ability to carry out these essential functions is hindered. Lack of sleep also causes our body to perceive stress; this elevates cortisol levels, which in turn triggers inflammation, wreaking havoc on our skin's integrity by breaking down collagen. Plus, when you're tired, the blood in your body is not flowing as efficiently. This causes the blood to have a reduced supply of oxygen, which is needed for proper collagen production.

The best way to ensure that you're getting quality sleep every night is to practice sleep hygiene. Think of sleep hygiene as self-care for your sleep. It consists of adjusting certain practices and environmental factors that affect your sleep to ensure that you're getting the best possible night's rest. Some of my best sleep hygiene tips include having a nightly routine to help you wind down before bed. Wear blue-light blocking glasses in the evening and avoid screens for at least an hour before bed. Avoid having a large meal right before bed to allow your body time to digest prior to sleeping. Sleep in a cool room without additional light and use aromatherapy to help you relax.

Smoking

We all know by now that smoking negatively affects your health. Quitting smoking should be at the top of your to-do list, if not for any other reason except vanity. According to a study by Insilico Medicine, a biotechnology company, smokers appeared to be twice as old as their chronological age when compared to nonsmokers.

Tobacco smoke has more than 4,000 chemicals that damage both collagen and elastin by elevating levels of oxidative stress from free radicals, which activates inflammatory responses and causes cellular damage. The nicotine in tobacco also narrows the blood vessels in the outer layers of the skin, reducing the delivery of nutrients and oxygen to the skin. Together, these processes accelerate the formation of wrinkles and loss of elasticity in the skin. Smoking also depletes the body of important antioxidants, such as vitamin C, that are needed for collagen production. To protect your skin from accelerated aging, do not smoke and do your best to avoid being around secondhand smoke.

Pollution

Air pollution and other environmental toxins can speed up the aging process and the breakdown of collagen. A landmark study in the *Journal of Investigative Dermatology* compared women living in urban and rural environments over a period of twenty-four years and found that those exposed to increased pollution had more dark spots and wrinkling. The toxin overload from pollution causes an increase in free radicals and in oxidative stress, a physiological type of stress that ages our cells. (Remember, stress in all forms contributes to the aging process and to the breakdown of collagen.) Oxidative stress causes collagen fibers to become fragmented and weak. As this happens, the body shifts into overdrive in an attempt to eliminate the free radicals, which depletes the important antioxidants that are necessary for proper collagen production.

To protect your skin against pollution, make simple changes: Properly cleanse your skin and increase the level of antioxidants in both your food and your skincare products. Wash your face to help flush the pores of dirt and other environmental pollutants that have penetrated the skin. And focus on antioxidant-rich foods and skincare products with ingredients such as vitamin C and vitamin E, which can have a significant impact on your skin.

Nutrient Deficiencies

As mentioned earlier, many nutrients play a supporting role in collagen production. A deficiency in any of these nutrients can limit collagen production and accelerate collagen loss. Eat a well-balanced diet that consists of nutrient-dense whole foods in the form of protein, healthy fats, fiber-rich carbohydrates, and antioxidants from fruits and vegetables. I cover the specific nutrients that play a role in collagen production in detail on pages 20–25.

Free-Radical Damage

Free-radical damage can come from many factors, including stress, pollution, and a lack of antioxidants in your diet. No matter where they come from, free radicals damage collagen fibers. Antioxidants that our body naturally produces, along with those we get from our diet, such as vitamin C, vitamin E, and carotenoids like beta-carotene, can protect us from free radicals. These antioxidants counteract the damage caused by free radicals and promote healthy cellular turnover. Think of antioxidants as free-radical scavengers, eating them all up like a cellular Pac-Man and reducing oxidative stress in the body.

Autoimmune Disorders

Some autoimmune disorders cause antibodies to target collagen. These disorders include lupus, rheumatoid arthritis, scleroderma, and temporal arteritis. Some individuals are born with disorders. For others, a trigger sets off an autoimmune condition later in life. Having an autoimmune condition can make it far more difficult to avoid collagen loss, but eating healthfully and using stress reduction techniques can decrease the chances of triggering immune responses or causing a flare-up of symptoms. If you have any medical conditions, it's important to talk with your doctor before making any diet or lifestyle changes.

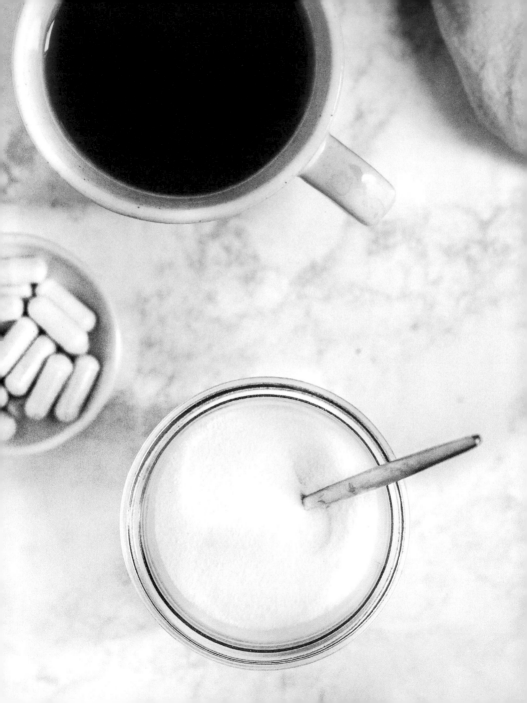

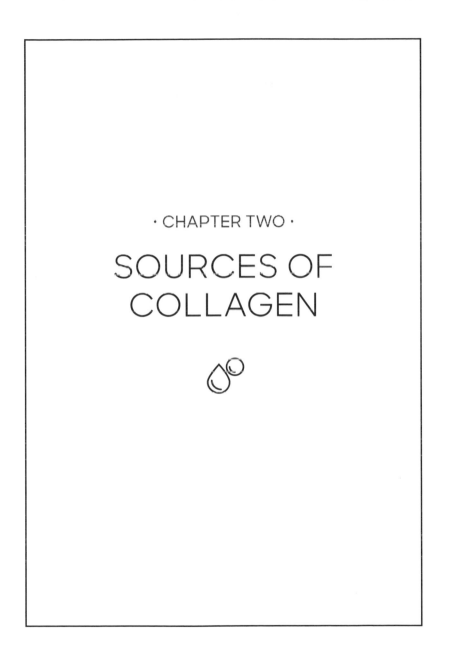

· CHAPTER TWO ·

SOURCES OF COLLAGEN

The only food sources of collagen come from animals. Some foods that contain collagen are the skins of chicken and fish, small fish bones, oxtails, liver, and chicken feet. To give you a better understanding of the whole-food sources of collagen, this list highlights the collagen-rich parts of beef, pork, chicken, fish, and egg that are used in collagen supplements.

Bovine collagen: This form of collagen is derived from cows. The cowhide, tendons, bones, cartilage, ligaments, bone marrow, and connective tissue are the main sources of collagen. Bovine collagen is rich in type I and type III collagen. Most bovine collagen supplements include collagen extracted from the bones and hide.

Porcine collagen: This type of collagen is derived from pigs. Like bovine collagen, porcine collagen comes primarily from the skin, tendons, bones, cartilage, ligaments, bone marrow, and connective tissue. Porcine collagen is rich in type I and type III collagen. Most gelatin is made from porcine collagen, which is extracted from bones and skin.

Aviary collagen: This form of collagen is derived from chicken. The main sources of collagen in chicken are the bones, cartilage, and tissues. Aviary collagen is rich in type II collagen, and most aviary collagen supplements come from cartilage.

Marine collagen: This type of collagen is derived from fish, specifically the fish skin, scales, bones, and cartilage. Marine collagen is slightly more bioavailable than the other types of collagen, meaning it's easier for your body to absorb because of the small size of the collagen peptides. Marine collagen is rich in type I collagen. Most marine collagen supplements use fish skins as their primary source of collagen.

Egg collagen: This type of collagen is found in the membrane between the eggshell and the egg white, which is rich in type I and type V collagen. The actual egg white and yolk contain a very small amount of collagen. Most egg-white collagen supplements use egg membrane as their main source of collagen.

As you can see, the collagen-rich parts of the animal are structural components, such as the skin, hide, and cartilage, which are tough and fibrous. You might assume you're getting enough collagen if you incorporate animal proteins like chicken, beef, eggs, and fish into your diet. Leaving the skin on chicken or fish or enjoying a bowl of pho may seem like easy ways to consume more collagen. Though you'll receive a small dose of collagen from these foods, collagen is most abundant in the skin, connective tissues, bones, and organ meat of animals; it's not as available in the lean muscle that most people are accustomed to eating. In addition, removing the skin from poultry and fish and choosing lean cuts of meat reduces your intake of the saturated fats and unhealthy inflammatory oils that are often used to make the skins flavorful and crispy. Although animal proteins can be part of a healthy diet, I encourage you to reduce your meat and animal protein consumption altogether for both health and environmental reasons.

This is why I recommend incorporating collagen supplements. They make it easy to consume collagen on a daily basis. You get all the benefits of collagen found in food without having to consume the whole animal. We'll learn more about supplements in chapter three.

COLLAGEN'S SUPPORTING NUTRIENTS

In addition to collagen-rich foods, there are several nutrients that play a supporting role in collagen production. Your body works hard to keep up with collagen production, and these vitamins and minerals keep this process going.

Vitamins and Minerals

These vitamins and minerals help the body build new collagen and protect its existing collagen from damage and deterioration.

Vitamin C

Vitamin C is the most well-known collagen supporter thanks to its prominent role in collagen production. It activates iron molecules and enzymes, creating links that stabilize collagen's triple-stranded helix shape. If you don't get enough vitamin C, this process can't run efficiently, which will cause your collagen production to slow. In addition, vitamin C acts as an antioxidant that fights free radicals in the body that are associated with aging and with exposure to UV light and pollutants. Both topical and food sources of vitamin C have been shown to help with collagen production.

Top food sources: bell peppers, berries, broccoli, brussels sprouts, cauliflower, citrus fruits (oranges, grapefruit, lemons, and limes), kale, and tropical fruits (mango, pineapple, papaya, kiwi, and guava)

Vitamin A

Vitamin A from both topical and food sources plays a vital role in collagen production and maintenance. Vitamin A signals to the cells to produce procollagen, the precursor to collagen. Topical vitamin A in the form of retinol stimulates collagen production and can be used as a treatment for antiaging and sun-damaged skin. Research also shows that carotenoids, which are precursors of vitamin A, can slow aging-related collagen breakdown.

Top food sources: cheese, eggs, and meat; plant-based foods that are high in carotenoids, include butternut squash, carrots, dried apricots, kale, pumpkin, sweet potatoes, and yellow and orange bell peppers

Iron

A small amount of iron is needed for collagen production. Like vitamin C, iron is part of the reaction that creates the links that stabilize collagen's triple-stranded helix shape. If you don't have enough iron, this process can't run efficiently, causing your collagen production to slow.

Top food sources: animal proteins and shellfish, blackstrap molasses, broccoli, kale, legumes, pumpkin seeds, quinoa, spinach, tahini, and tofu

Zinc

Zinc is commonly used in hospitals as a treatment for burns, certain ulcers, and other skin injuries because of the important role it plays in collagen production, immune function, and inflammatory response. Zinc activates the proteins responsible for making collagen. Without enough zinc, the cross-links that give strength and structure to collagen molecules are impaired. Zinc is also a key nutrient in the function of collagenase, which allows your cells to remodel collagen after damage. This is especially important during wound healing.

Top food sources: cacao powder, cashews, chickpeas, dairy products, fish, meat, poultry, and pumpkin seeds

Copper

It's been shown that copper increases the production of collagen, especially types I, II, and V. Copper activates an enzyme called lysyl oxidase that's required for collagen maturation. Active lysyl oxidase cross-links collagen fibers that further stabilize mature collagen and help to form the scaffolding that supports the tissues in the body.

Top food sources: almonds, blackstrap molasses, cacao powder, cashews, dried prunes, kale, lentils, oysters, sesame seeds, shiitake mushrooms, and sunflower seeds

Silicon (Silica)

Silicon is a naturally occurring mineral that is an essential component of collagen and other connective tissues, such as elastin. It's thought to play both a metabolic and a structural role. A lack of silicon in the body causes a decrease in an enzyme required for collagen formation and increased collagen breakdown.

Top food sources: artichokes, brown rice, burdock, green beans, mangoes, horseradish, oatmeal, spinach, and whole grains

Nutraceuticals and Herbs

This wide variety of plant extracts, herbs, and nutrients can help boost healthy collagen production in the body.

Phytoceramides

Phytoceramides are waxy lipid molecules derived from plants. These plant-based molecules perform the same functions as the ceramides that are naturally found in high concentrations within our cell membranes. Phytoceramides from the foods we eat travel to new skin cells through the bloodstream; they help the skin retain moisture, smooth wrinkles, and support collagen production. We naturally lose ceramides, just as we lose collagen, as we age. Research shows that women between thirty and sixty years old with dry skin saw improvements in skin elasticity, reduction in micro-wrinkles, and an increase in skin smoothness when they ingested 70 milligrams of phytoceramides daily for eight weeks.

Top food sources: brown rice, dairy, eggs, soybeans, spinach, sweet potatoes, and wheat germ

Astaxanthin

Astaxanthin is a carotenoid that occurs naturally in microalgae and seafood like salmon. This is what gives algae, salmon, shrimp, and other foods their natural red, yellow, and green hues. Astaxanthin is a powerful antioxidant with sixty-five times more antioxidant potential than vitamin C. Because of its antioxidant abilities, it can help fight free radicals that cause collagen breakdown. One study looked at the combination of astaxanthin and collagen hydrolysate supplementation on moderately photoaged skin. Forty-four participants consumed 2 milligrams of astaxanthin combined with 3 grams of collagen hydrolysate or placebos daily for twelve weeks. The results showed that astaxanthin combined with collagen hydrolysate improved elasticity and reduced water loss in their photoaged skin. It also resulted in a decrease in the gene expression associated with slowing the breakdown of existing collagen.

Top food sources: algae, crayfish, krill, salmon, shrimp, trout, and yeast

Hyaluronic Acid

Hyaluronic acid is a substance found in almost every cell in our body, but largely in the skin, connective tissue, and eyes. Its main function is to keep your skin hydrated and tissues well lubricated with its ability to retain 1,000 times its own weight in water. Since hyaluronic acid can retain so much moisture, it's often used in skincare products. However, it's also an effective supplement that has been shown to help aging skin, osteoarthritis, dry eyes, and wound healing. Hyaluronic acid and collagen are a dream team, especially for the skin and joints. While collagen firms the skin, hyaluronic acid hydrates the collagen by holding on to water. Together, they help keep the skin hydrated, reducing the appearance of fine lines and wrinkles, accelerating wound healing, and relieving joint pain in people with osteoarthritis.

Top food sources: almonds, bananas, bone broth, Japanese sweet potatoes, leafy greens, meat, and seafood

ADDITIONAL COLLAGEN BOOSTERS

There are quite a few other nutrients and plants that are well-known collagen supporters. Thanks to their antioxidant properties, many of these supporters help increase collagen production and reduce its breakdown.

- Algae (spirulina)
- Amla
- Burdock
- Chlorophyll
- Cinnamon
- Coenzyme Q10
- Ginseng
- Gotu kola
- Grape skin extract
- Green tea
- Labisia pumila
- Luteolin
- Marigold
- Omega-3s
- Selenium
- Sulfur

Even though some have a more prominent role than others, the number of nutrients and plant extracts in this list shows the complexity of our bodies and the collagen process. For example, many of the plant extracts act as antioxidants that help reverse the damage to collagen from aging, the sun, pollution, or any of the other collagen killers. This is a long list (and it's far from a complete list of all of the collagen supporters), so I encourage you to focus on getting the main nutrients described on pages 20-24 through your diet. You don't need to incorporate all of the supporters to build and maintain collagen.

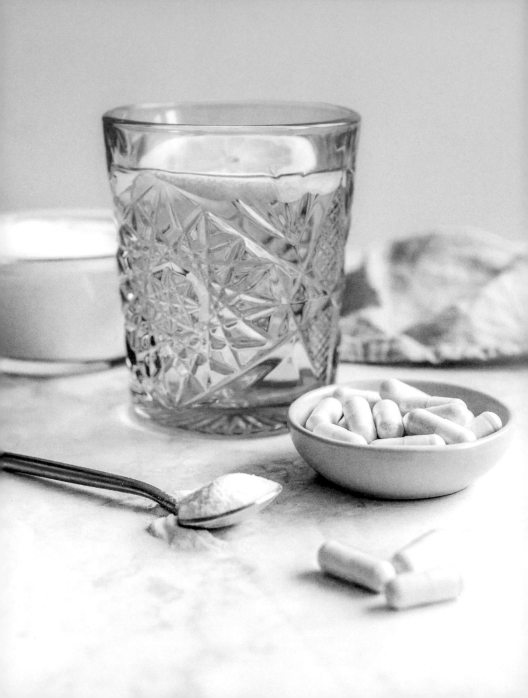

· CHAPTER THREE ·

COLLAGEN
SUPPLEMENTS

I strongly encourage focusing on eating foods in their most natural form, but collagen is an exception. You'll benefit more from incorporating a collagen supplement than from trying to get all your daily collagen through whole-food sources. Supplements enable you to incorporate collagen into your daily routine without having to always rely on eating animal protein or the collagen-rich parts of the animal like the skin, tendons, or cartilage.

Collagen supplements can boost your protein intake and help you reach your daily protein needs. Even though it's not considered a complete protein because it's missing the essential amino acid tryptophan, it gives you many of the essential amino acids you need to get through your diet. And when paired with other protein from plant-based or animal protein sources consumed throughout the day, you can be sure that you are getting all the amino acids needed to create the protein and collagen your body needs to thrive.

THE BENEFITS OF COLLAGEN SUPPLEMENTS

We know now that collagen provides the structure and support for skin, hair, nails, joints, and other connective tissues like cartilage and tendons. Since collagen is found throughout the entire body, it's no wonder the benefits are widespread.

Before we dive into all the amazing benefits of collagen supplements, I want to acknowledge that there are many skeptics. This is completely understandable! Research on collagen supplementation is still a very new science and is still limited, since it's a fairly new topic of study. Quality studies can take years, even decades, to provide long-term results. It also doesn't help that companies make inaccurate claims or market collagen as the "fountain of youth" for every ailment.

As of 2019, the majority of research has focused on the benefits of collagen supplements for skin, joint, and bone health. However, new research is emerging on the role of collagen supplements in gut health and digestion, weight loss and satiety, muscle gain and recovery, and wound healing. Other research also looks at the benefits of glycine and proline, the main amino acids in collagen, and collagen as a protein source. As a registered dietitian, I have the job of digging deep into the science available now while also being open-minded moving into the future. From all my research, I can confidently say there are incredible benefits that arise from taking collagen supplements. Let's dive into the main science-backed ones.

COLLAGEN BENEFITS
- Improves skin elasticity
- Increases skin hydration
- Increases skin firmness
- Reduces the appearance of cellulite
- Strengthens nails
- Thickens hair
- Maintains strong bones
- Protects against osteoporosis
- Improves joint health
- Heals gut lining
- Improves digestion
- Accelerates muscle gain and recovery
- Increases satiety
- Aids in weight loss
- Promotes wound healing

Skin

Our skin is the largest organ of the body, containing more than 40 percent of the body's collagen. It's the protective layer around our entire body and acts as a strong but flexible barrier protecting the body from impact, moisture, temperature changes, and germs and toxic substances. Collagen is one of the skin's main structural components and helps with elasticity and hydration. Together, these qualities provide taut, glowing, youthful-looking skin. As our collagen production starts to decline with age and lifestyle habits, we start to notice saggy skin, wrinkles, more pronounced cellulite, and an all-around lackluster appearance.

The most well-known benefit of collagen supplementation is its antiaging effect on the skin. Some claim that collagen makes the skin look tighter and gives it a smoother appearance and that sought-after glow. This may be the most popular reason for consuming collagen, but there are many other claims about benefits, ranging from improving joint health to facilitating weight loss to healing the gut. But what does the science say?

Numerous double-blind studies showcase the benefits of collagen for skin elasticity, firmness, and hydration, all of which can help keep skin looking younger and prevent accelerated signs of aging. Several other studies have shown that taking collagen peptides or supplements containing collagen may reduce wrinkles and dryness. The wrinkle-reducing effects of collagen supplements have been attributed to the supplements' ability to stimulate your body's production of collagen. It's been shown that taking collagen supplements may promote the production of elastin and fibrillin, which are other proteins that help provide structure for your skin.

In one double-blind study, 214 women between the ages of twenty-five and forty-five were divided into five groups and instructed to consume 2.5 grams, 5 grams, or 10 grams of collagen peptides from fish scales daily for four weeks. Moisture content significantly increased for groups that consumed 5 grams or 10 grams of collagen peptides. In another double-blind study of sixty-nine women between the ages of thirty-five and fifty five, the participants were given 2.5 grams or 5 grams of collagen peptides daily for eight weeks. The results showed that skin elasticity improved at weeks 4 and 8 compared with the placebo group. In addition, the skin's moisture content improved in women fifty years or older. A placebo-controlled trial found that supplementing with 10 grams of collagen peptides for eight weeks significantly improved skin hydration and increased collagen density in the skin. The trial also found that collagen supplementation reduced collagen breakdown in the skin.

I can't talk about collagen and skin without mentioning cellulite. This dimpled appearance is thought of as less desirable, but in reality it is the norm. It's estimated that less than 15 percent of women don't have cellulite. Cellulite is a condition in which the skin has a dimpled, lumpy appearance. It usually affects the buttocks and thighs but can also occur in other areas. Cellulite occurs when fat deposits push through the connective tissue beneath the skin. We all have a layer of fat deposit underneath the skin. When the collagen in the connective tissue weakens, the fat protrudes through the weakened tissue, giving the skin a dimpled appearance. As we age, our skin becomes thinner and loses elasticity, largely because of the loss of collagen; this increases the chances that cellulite will appear. Weakening tissues along with genetics and other changes, such as a slower metabolism, a more sedentary lifestyle, muscle loss, and hormone shifts that come with age, all play a role as well. From age twenty-five to thirty-five, right when collagen production starts declining, you might start seeing more cellulite. Cellulite also becomes more pronounced as women reach menopause and estrogen starts decreasing, which in turn decreases collagen production. When estrogen starts to decrease, you lose receptors in blood vessels, especially in the thighs and buttocks, which decreases circulation and allows less oxygen and nutrition to flow to that area.

Research shows that collagen supplements may help. One study found a reduction in cellulite in women who took bioactive collagen peptides. This was a double-blind, placebo-controlled clinical study that administered bioactive collagen peptides to over a period of six months women ages twenty-four through fifty who had moderate cellulite at healthy or unhealthy weights. The results indicated that the women who received 2.5 grams of bioactive collagen peptides experienced a statistically significant decrease in the degree of cellulite, and those with normal weights saw a reduction in skin waviness on their thighs. The collagen treatment also had similar effects for overweight women, although the impact was less pronounced.

What about other skin conditions, like acne and eczema? There are anecdotal claims that collagen supplements are helpful for preventing acne and other skin conditions, but these are not yet supported by scientific studies. If you're struggling with a skin condition, taking collagen supplements may help. However, it's important to talk with your doctor before starting a new supplement regimen for any medical condition.

Hair and Nails

Take one look at the beauty industry and it's clear that beautiful hair and nails are in high demand. What is considered healthy when it comes to hair and nails? Healthy hair is typically defined as shiny and voluminous and not dull, brittle, splitting, or excessively shedding. Healthy nails can be described similarly: they shouldn't be brittle, peeling, splitting, bending, or discolored.

As we age, collagen production slows, causing hair and nails to become brittle and weak. This may come as a surprise because your hair and nails are made not of collagen, but of keratin. Like collagen, keratin consists of three strands of amino acid chains that are twisted into a triple helix. However, the amino acid sequence in keratin is very different from the one in collagen, making it much stronger and more resistant to breakdown. This gives our hair and nails their structure and incredible strength.

Though collagen is not directly located in hair and nails, some studies show that it can hydrate them, helping them grow faster and thicker. Proline, one of the main amino acids in keratin, is also found in collagen. When you consume proline-rich collagen, you're providing your body with the building blocks it needs to create new hair and nails.

Several studies suggest that ingesting collagen supports healthy hair A study published in the *Journal of Investigative Dermatology* found that there are large collagen deposits in hair follicles. The findings of this study suggest the existence of "essential relationships between extracellular matrix (ECM) and hair follicle regeneration, suggesting that collagen benefits could include being a potential therapeutic target for hair loss and other skin-related diseases."

Another study found that consuming 14 grams of collagen-rich gelatin daily increased the average diameter of individual hair strands by 9 to 11 percent, with some experiencing a 45 percent increase. Six months after participants had stopped consuming gelatin, their hair diameters went back to their original levels, showcasing how important daily ingestion of collagen-rich gelatin was for maintaining hair thickness for study participants.

As far as research on nails goes, a few small studies show how collagen supplements can benefit nails. One study found that consuming 5 grams of collagen peptides daily for twelve weeks prevented drying and improved nail flexibility in women who had trouble with thin, fragile nails that peeled off. The nails had improved moisture retention because of an increase in sphingosine and ceramide, intercellular lipids (also known as the fat molecules found inside the cells) in the nails.

Another small study found that consuming 2.5 grams of bioactive collagen peptides once daily for twenty-four weeks increased nail growth and decreased nail brittleness and breakage. The nail growth rate increased by 12 percent, and the frequency of broken nails decreased by 42 percent. The only downsides of this study were that it included only 25 participants and lacked a control group. Clearly, more research is needed in the area of collagen and nail health, but these studies point toward promising results.

Bone Health

When talking about bone health, calcium and vitamin D are the main nutrients that come to mind. These nutrients, along with other minerals, do play an important role. However, 80 percent of all the protein in bone is made of type I collagen, which gives your bones structure and helps with their strength and resiliency. Since bones hold an abundant amount of collagen, you can imagine why many believe that collagen supplements can help maintain bone health and guard against osteoporosis.

With age, collagen production slows and deterioration accelerates. The same is true for bone mineral density. Bone mineral density is a measure of the amount of minerals, such as calcium and phosphorus, in your bones. Low bone mineral density is associated with weak bones and may lead to conditions such as osteoporosis, which is linked to a higher risk of bone fractures.

So far, a few studies have shown that taking collagen supplements may help reduce the accelerated bone breakdown that leads to osteoporosis. In one study, thirty-nine osteopenic postmenopausal women took either a calcium–vitamin D supplement combined with

5 grams of collagen or a calcium–vitamin D supplement and no collagen daily for twelve months. By the end of the study, the women taking the calcium–vitamin D supplement combined with collagen had significantly lower blood levels of proteins that promote bone breakdown than those taking only the calcium–vitamin D. These results highlight that the combination of collagen with the calcium–vitamin D supplement was beneficial for reducing bone loss in osteopenic postmenopausal women.

Another double-blind, controlled study found similar results in sixty-six women who took 5 grams of supplemental collagen daily for twelve months. The postmenopausal women who took the collagen had up to a 7 percent greater increase in their bone mineral density than did women who did not consume collagen. The results show a favorable shift in bone markers indicating increased bone formation and reduced bone degradation.

Since bone loss is an inevitable part of the aging process, incorporating diet and lifestyle changes that can slow this process is extremely important for aging well. Weight-bearing exercise, hormonal balance, adequate sleep, and getting enough of the nutrients that are essential for bone health, such as vitamin D, calcium, magnesium, and zinc, can all help slow bone loss. Adequate protein is also important for maintaining bone health. Although a few studies showcase the benefits of collagen for bone health, the jury is still out. More human studies are needed, especially in nonorthopedic women and men, but collagen supplements can easily help you reach the daily protein intake needed for healthy bones.

Joint Health

Healthy joints are well-cushioned and move properly without pain. As we age, joint pain can start to become more noticeable as the cartilage found in the joints starts to wear down. This is where collagen supplements can help.

Today, most of the research on collagen supplements focuses on joint health, because collagen is a major component of cartilage found in the joints. In the United States, osteoarthritis affects more than twenty-five million Americans. This type of arthritis destroys joint cartilage and causes remodeling of the adjacent bone. Current therapies for osteoarthritis include various over-the-counter painkillers, nonsteroidal anti-inflammatory drugs (NSAIDs), and injections of corticosteroids or hyaluronic acid, to name just a few. However, these treatments come with potential side effects. Collagen supplements, on the other hand, have very little risk and have been shown to benefit those with joint issues, including osteoarthritis.

Research on collagen supplements and joint health shows that collagen may help maintain the integrity of cartilage, improve symptoms of osteoarthritis, and reduce joint pain. It's thought that the amino acids from ingested collagen stimulate the synthesis of new collagen in the cartilage and other tissues in the joints. Most of the research on collagen and joint health uses a unique type of collagen known as undenatured type II collagen (UC-II), which is derived from chicken sternum cartilage. This differs from most other types of collagen used in research in that it's not broken down into highly absorbable collagen peptides. Many clinical studies suggest that the ingestion of 10 grams of UC-II per day for three months results in reduced pain and improvement in joint function.

Another clinical trial showed that UC-II consumption was a better treatment option than glucosamine and chondroitin supplements for osteoarthritis of the knee. Of the fifty participants, one half took 40 milligrams of undenatured collagen type II and the other half took 1,500 milligrams of glucosamine and 1,200 milligrams of chondroitin daily. The results indicated that UC-II was two to three times more effective in reducing pain than the combination of glucosamine and chondroitin and significantly improved patients' ability to go about daily activities, thereby improving their quality of life.

Research has also been conducted on collagen supplements and the joint health of athletes. One double-blind, placebo-controlled study conducted at Penn State University studied 147 athletes over the course of twenty-four weeks. Seventy-three athletes consumed 10 grams of collagen hydrolysate daily, and the other seventy-four athletes consumed a placebo. The results showed that the seventy-three athletes who consumed the collagen experienced a significant decrease in joint pain while walking and at rest compared to a group that did not take it.

These are just a few of the studies that showcase the benefits of collagen supplements in relation to joint health. Although many beneficial results have been attained, more research should be conducted on the long-term effects of different types of collagen in relation to joint health in healthy adults, athletes, and those with osteoarthritis.

Gut Lining and Digestive Health

A healthy digestive system is important for optimal health. Your digestive system affects many body processes, from your ability to digest food and absorb nutrients to how well your metabolism and immune system work. Despite the importance of a healthy gut, food sensitivities, irritable bowel syndrome (IBS), and other digestive issues are on the rise. Numerous factors, such as stress, autoimmune diseases, pain meds, infections, toxins, gluten, and overexercising, can lead to a compromised gut lining. These stressors can damage the collagen-rich tissue lining the intestinal tract, causing "leaky gut" or intestinal permeability. The tight junctions between the cells of the intestinal tract loosen, allowing bacteria and other toxins to leak out of your small intestine and into your bloodstream, triggering an inflammatory reaction, gut inflammation, and malabsorption of nutrients. Intestinal permeability is now thought to be the basis for many digestive conditions, including infectious enterocolitis, inflammatory bowel disease (IBD), small intestinal bacterial overgrowth (SIBO), celiac disease, irritable bowel syndrome (IBS), hepatic fibrosis, food intolerances, and skin conditions.

If you want to achieve optimal health, you need to have a gut lining that is strong and uncompromised. Collagen supplements have been shown to improve digestion and the health of the gut lining. Since collagen is the main component in the lining of your intestinal wall, collagen supplements provide your body with an excellent source of the amino acids needed to rebuild the rapidly dividing cells that line the gut. Research shows that supplementing with specific amino acids, including arginine, glutamine, glutamate, threonine, methionine, serine, and proline, can support the healing of the gut lining. In addition, glutamine is key for preventing gut inflammation and reducing oxidative stress in the intestines. Since collagen's main amino acids are glycine and proline, collagen supplements are an easy way to get those beneficial amino acids. They also contain a good amount of glutamic acid, which is converted to glutamine in the body.

Collagen is well tolerated and easily digested, making it especially helpful to those with compromised digestive systems that are easily irritated. In addition, the structural properties and amino acid profile of collagen can reduce gut inflammation, heal stomach ulcers, aid digestion, and regulate stomach acid secretion. Gelatin provides additional benefits to digestive health through its ability to attract water. Gelatin also helps keep fluid in the digestive tract and creates a protective coating on the intestinal lining. This can help with overall digestion in healthy individuals, but it is especially beneficial for those with digestive issues. Recent studies have highlighted using gelatin as a gut-lining protector as a way to manage intestinal diseases and restore the gut barrier.

In addition to helping to restore and maintain the integrity of your interior gut lining, collagen may help your stomach lining. Collagen is rich in glycine and proline, the main amino acids found in the stomach lining, which have been shown to be helpful in healing the stomach lining and preventing stress-induced ulcers. The abundance of glycine in collagen can help reduce acid reflux and gastroesophageal reflux disease (GERD), since glycine assists with digestion and with reducing gastric acid secretion.

It is important to mention that research on digestive health and the microbiome in relation to collagen is still in its infancy. Most studies have looked at the effects of isolated amino acids in a clinical setting. More research is needed on collagen supplements and their benefits for gut health.

Muscle Gain and Recovery

Protein is extremely important for building and maintaining muscle. Without adequate protein, muscles start to break down, especially as we age. Around the age of thirty, most men and women experience a 3 to 8 percent decrease in muscle every decade, a condition known as sarcopenia. We start to lose muscle as we age for many reasons, but decreasing testosterone levels in men and decreasing estrogen levels in women are main contributors to muscle loss. The aging body also converts amino acids to muscle tissue less efficiently. Muscle loss isn't necessarily inevitable. Adults can maintain and build muscles as they age by incorporating regular resistance training exercises and making sure they are meeting their nutrient requirements for protein, carbohydrates, and healthy fats.

Collagen supplements have been shown to help build muscle, reduce exercise-induced inflammation, and repair tissue by supplying the body with some of the amino acids necessary for building muscle and for tissue repair. A few studies have shown collagen supplements to be extremely beneficial for boosting muscle mass in people with sarcopenia. One double-blind, placebo-controlled study looked at the effect of collagen as a post-exercise protein supplement following resistance training in elderly subjects with sarcopenia. Fifty-three elderly men with sarcopenia were split into two groups. For twelve weeks, one group consumed 15 grams of collagen peptides per day, while the other group took a placebo. All the participants underwent a twelve-week guided resistance training program with three training sessions per week. All study participants increased their muscle mass, bone mass, and quadriceps strength, and they all reduced their body fat. However, the participants given collagen peptides had a greater increase in muscle mass and a greater reduction in body fat. The researchers speculated that collagen's high levels of glycine and arginine, amino acids that the body converts into the muscle-building compound creatinine, produced these results.

One very small double-blind, placebo-controlled pilot study explored whether BioCell Collagen®, which is a supplement made from hydrolyzed chicken cartilage, could improve recovery from intense exercise for eight healthy, active individuals with an average age of twenty-nine years old. The participants were split into two groups and given either 3 grams of BioCell Collagen or 3 grams of a placebo for six weeks. After six weeks of supplementation, the participants performed upper-body resistance exercises designed to result in muscle damage and repeated these same exercises three days later. During each of the two exercise sessions, the individuals who took the collagen had lower blood markers for muscle tissue damage and were able to perform more repetitions than the placebo group. Again, one reason younger, healthy adults may see beneficial results regarding collagen supplements and muscle gain may be the high concentration of the amino acid glycine in this protein.

The present research shows that collagen supplements can be somewhat beneficial for muscle gain and recovery. That being said, I recommend incorporating a wide variety of protein sources into your diet, while aiming for 20–40 grams of protein per meal, for optimal muscle gain. High-protein foods are very important for gaining muscle, but you can't just eat protein and expect to gain muscle. Carbohydrates and fats are also necessary sources of energy and are essential for recovery. Remember, collagen is not a complete protein, so it should not be used as the only source of protein throughout the day. If you're using powdered collagen as a protein powder replacement, you need to ingest other quality protein sources throughout the day to ensure that you're getting all the amino acids you need and in the right quantities for optimal muscle-building and recovery.

Weight Loss and Satiety

Many companies claim, as a marketing strategy, that collagen supplements can help you lose weight. As a registered dietitian, I can confidently tell you that there is no one food or ingredient that is going to drastically help you lose weight. There is no magic ingredient or simple weight-loss equation. Gone are the days of weight loss being a direct effect of eating fewer calories than you burn. Although the amount you eat matters, the quality of food, hormones, sleep, hunger cues, exercise, gut health, genetics, and your own unique build all play a role.

Claims that collagen promotes weight loss largely call on the fact that it's a protein. Out of all the macronutrients, protein provides the most satiety. This means that eating protein keeps you full longer than if you were eating just carbohydrates or fat. Research shows that individuals who increased protein consumption and consumed fewer glycemic foods had more significant weight loss and maintained weight loss longer than those eating diets with less protein. (This is why I always recommend incorporating protein into every meal and snack. It will help keep you satisfied, reduce cravings, and prevent overeating.)

In another small study, twenty-four healthy adults participated in research looking at the satiety effects of various protein supplements. For breakfast, the participants were given a custard made from one of seven different types of protein: casein, soy, whey, whey without glycomacropeptide, alpha-lactalbumin (a protein derived from dairy), gelatin, or gelatin with tryptophan. The results showed that alpha-lactalbumin, gelatin, and gelatin with tryptophan were found to be 40 percent more satiating than the other types of protein. The participants who got those forms of protein ended up eating 20 percent fewer calories at lunch. The researchers concluded that gelatin increases satiety, which can subsequently reduce caloric intake and help promote weight loss.

A similar study involving participants who consumed only one type of protein found that a gelatin diet suppressed appetite 44 percent more than a diet made up of only casein, a common dairy protein. However, one downside was that consuming only gelatin caused the participants to lose a small amount of body protein, which could contribute to loss of muscle mass over time. This wasn't a surprise, since gelatin is not a complete protein and all essential amino acids are needed to support muscle growth and maintenance. This study showcased that even though gelatin can help suppress hunger hormones, it can't constitute the sole source of protein in the diet and should be used in conjunction with complete sources of protein.

The research on collagen supplements and weight loss is slim, and all the existing studies involve small populations. However, collagen supplements can be used along with other dietary and lifestyle changes needed to promote weight loss. Just make sure not to discount other factors that can help you maintain a healthy weight, including hormones, sleep, hunger cues, exercise, and gut health.

Wound Healing

Collagen is rich in glycine and proline, amino acids that are conditionally essential during times of stress. The need for these amino acids is even more pronounced when healing from a wound. Proline and glycine help regenerate cartilage, which forms connective tissue and repairs wounds. Research shows that the levels of proline in a wound are at least 50 percent higher than those in the blood.

Studies have shown that consuming collagen may speed wound healing. Several randomized controlled trials have found that collagen hydrolysate supplement results in individuals with pressure ulcers (also known as bedsores) recovering significantly faster than if they received only standard care. There isn't much research yet on the impact of collagen supplements on less severe wounds, but we do know that ingesting collagen can help ensure that your body has a constant supply of proline and glycine in case it needs to use them for repair and recovery.

DIFFERENT TYPES OF COLLAGEN SUPPLEMENTS

Collagen supplements come in a variety of forms. No matter what your daily routine or eating style looks like, there is a collagen supplement for you.

Collagen Peptides

Collagen peptides are my favorite way to supplement collagen. They take the form of a tasteless, odorless powder that can dissolve into almost any food or beverage, hot or cold. This makes them extremely easy to add to recipes.

What are collagen peptides? Remember that collagen is a very large protein molecule. As mentioned earlier, the main types of collagen (types I, II, and III) have three amino acid chains that coil into an incredibly tight triple-helix structure. This structure makes collagen very hard for our body to break down and absorb.

Collagen peptides are a broken-down version of collagen. Their small protein molecules are much more bioavailable. The final product has a molecular weight within the range of 500–25,000 daltons, which is extremely tiny. This results in collagen peptides that have a more than 90 percent absorption rate, which is three times more than the absorption rate of collagen in its whole-food form. The small size of the collagen peptide protein molecules means they can dissolve into almost any food or beverage without changing their consistency.

To break down the large collagen protein molecules into collagen peptides, the large collagen proteins undergo a process called hydrolysis. Hydrolysis is the breakdown of a compound that results from a reaction with water, which produces a broken hydrogen bond. Collagen can be hydrolyzed with chemicals or enzymes. Enzymes are typically preferred because they make it much easier to control the reaction without ruining the unique properties of the collagen. Hydrolysis is only one step in the process of turning collagen into absorbable collagen peptides. It also involves the extraction of the collagen-rich parts of the animal, such as tendons, skin, and bones, and boiling these animal tissues to transform the collagen to gelatin. This process includes enzymatic hydrolysis, filtration, evaporation, sterilization, and finally drying.

You may see supplements with the terms "collagen peptides," "hydrolyzed collagen," or "collagen hydrolysate." These names are interchangeable. They're all just a way of saying that the collagen has been broken down into convenient and easy-to-digest peptides using hydrolysis.

Gelatin

Collagen proteins that undergo partial hydrolysis are called gelatin. Unlike collagen peptides, gelatin is not broken down by enzymes. The breakdown is key for making collagen peptides soluble in both hot and cold liquids. Skipping it keeps the hydrogen bonds between the strands of amino acids. These larger molecules are too big to dissolve in cold water, so gelatin is soluble easily only in hot liquids.

Since gelatin has to be dissolved in hot water, it's best used as a thickener or in desserts like ice cream, pudding, or gummies, where it can give food a smooth, creamy texture. When the dissolved gelatin comes into contact with cold liquid, it solidifies (think of gelatin desserts, marshmallows, custards, and gummies).

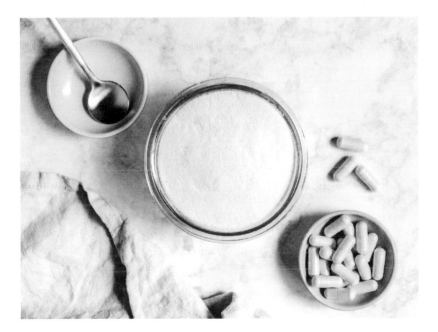

These unique properties of gelatin contribute to some of its gut-healing properties. Like other forms of collagen, it's rich in the amino acids glycine, proline, and glutamine. These amino acids are necessary for improving gut integrity, and they decrease gut permeability and restore the stomach lining. Since gelatin is made up of bigger molecules than collagen peptides, it takes slightly longer to digest. It can also absorb water and gel, helping the digestive tract retain fluid and creating a soothing coating on the small intestine that can help keep things moving and encourages normal bowel movements. For these reasons, gelatin is one of the key components in gut-healing protocols like the GAPS (gut and psychology syndrome) diet and other elimination diets that are designed to heal the gut and promote healthy digestion.

Bone Broth

Bone broth is a collagen-rich liquid that is made by slowly simmering the bones and connective tissue of animals. Unlike stock, which is typically simmered for only a few hours, bone broth is often simmered for 24 to 72 hours to break down the bones and release as many nutrients and minerals as possible. The result is a nutritious broth that's filled with gelatin and various nutrients that are extracted from the bones while they're simmering. Consuming bone broth is a great way to enjoy the benefits of collagen. You can easily incorporate it into your diet by replacing your normal broth or stock with bone broth in soups, sauces, and gravies. You can also simply warm it on the stovetop with aromatics like ginger, onion, and garlic, and season it with salt, pepper, or other spices to have as a healing, mineral-rich drink.

The extra benefit of consuming bone broth rather than gelatin or collagen peptides is that the broth contains minerals from the bones and hyaluronic acid, which is found in the synovial fluid of the joints and skin.

Animal bones are rich in calcium, magnesium, potassium, phosphorus, and other trace minerals. These just happen to be the same minerals needed to strengthen your own bones. And because fish swim in iodine-rich seawater, they contain the added benefit of iodine, which is essential for a healthy metabolism and a well-functioning thyroid. The collagen-rich connective tissues are also full of glucosamine and chondroitin, natural compounds that are found in cartilage and known to support joint health. Last but not least, bone marrow provides vitamins A and K_2, minerals like zinc, iron, boron, manganese, and selenium, and fatty acids omega-3 and omega-6.

Unfortunately, it's impossible to know the exact amount of collagen and each nutrient in bone broth because the nutrition profile of each batch of bones can vary greatly depending on its source. It's best to make your own bone broth because you can control how long it simmers. Research has shown that homemade bone broth is a better source of collagen, amino acids, and nutrients than standardized recipes used for commercial production. If you are buying bone broth, make sure it's from a high-quality source and made from grass fed, pasture-raised, or wild-caught animals. It's also important to make sure the bone broth has been cooked for at least twelve hours and uses an acid like apple cider vinegar. This will ensure it's been cooked long enough for the nutrients to be extracted and for you to get the full benefits of the broth.

Capsules and Liquid Collagen

Capsules and liquid collagen are convenient because you don't have to add anything to a liquid or food in order to consume the collagen. You just have to remember to take it! If you already have a supplement regimen in place, adding a collagen supplement in capsule form may be easy. Most of the collagens in capsule form are collagen peptides. However, there are gelatin capsules as well.

Liquid collagen is taking off as another convenient way to get your daily dose of collagen. These products range from liquid tinctures that can be added to a liquid of your choice to premade collagen coffees and flavored waters. Since these products use hydrolyzed collagen peptides, the collagen dissolves completely in the liquid. However, many of these products are sweetened either with natural sugars, such as stevia or monk fruit, or with artificial sweeteners like sucralose.

Many collagen supplements that come in capsule or liquid form have additional nutrients or herbs to help support collagen production

SPOTLIGHT ON TOPICAL COLLAGEN

Until recently, collagen used to be found only in topical skin care products and injectables. However, ingestible collagen supplements are gaining in popularity for a reason. Most topical skin care products don't live up to their claims of increasing collagen production and reducing the appearance of dull skin, fine lines, and wrinkles. Traditional topical collagen products used nonhydrolyzed collagen protein. This type of collagen molecule is too big to penetrate the outer layer of your skin. That being said, new products contain hydrolyzed collagen, or collagen peptides. This type of collagen is able to make its way through the outer layer of the skin and penetrate into the dermis (or the middle layer of the skin), where it can help make new collagen. There isn't much research out there on topical collagen peptides and improved skin appearance, especially regarding long-term use. Still, you may find that collagen creams help moisturize the skin, making it feel softer and smoother. This is because well hydrated and moisturized skin looks less dull and might make wrinkles look less prominent.

or address other health concerns. You can find collagen supplements that target the skin and include nutrients like vitamin C, vitamin E, and hyaluronic acid. Other collagen supplements contain chondroitin sulfate to help support joint health. Depending on the concerns you want to address, you may find that a collagen capsule that has additional supporting nutrients is the best option for you.

Collagen-Enhanced Food Products

There are tons of collagen-packed products available on the shelves of health food stores and even mainstream supermarkets. Everything from

ARE COLLAGEN SUPPLEMENTS VEGAN?

You've probably realized by now that collagen supplements are not vegan. Since collagen is made only in humans and animals, there are currently no vegan sources of collagen. However, there are plant-based foods that are rich in vitamins, minerals, and antioxidants that can boost your body's natural collagen production (see pages 20–25), including almonds, spinach, kale, papaya, sweet potatoes, berries, lentils, and pumpkin seeds, to name just a few.

Making sure you're getting protein from a variety of plant foods throughout the day is important ensuring that your body has all the amino acids you need, including collagens, to build proteins. It's also important to make sure you are supporting your body with enough foods that are high in proline and glycine. These are the main amino acids needed to support collagen production. Vegan sources of proline and glycine include soy, beans, spinach, cabbage, cauliflower, avocados, asparagus, and sunflower seeds.

protein bars to gummies is getting loaded with collagen. Even water is getting a collagen boost!

When choosing one of these products, beware of ones that contain added sugars or other preservatives, artificial flavors, noncaloric sweeteners, or chemical additives. A lot of brands use these ingredients to enhance the taste of their products. If you are going to opt for a collagen-packed product, it's important to read the label. Look at the ingredient list and make sure you're familiar with each ingredient. If you don't know what an ingredient is, chances are your body won't know what it is either. For this reason, I do not typically recommend gummy collagen supplements. Most of the time, they are sugar based and have added ingredients and fillers.

When it comes down to it, you're always better off eating foods in their most natural form. Instead of loading up on an ultra-processed snack food just because it contains collagen, grab a to-go packet of collagen peptides and add it to your latte, or sip some bone broth.

USING COLLAGEN SUPPLEMENTS

Questions about taking collagen supplements arise frequently. This section addresses the most common ones.

How Do I Choose a Collagen Supplement?

Not all collagen is created equal. Since collagen is an animal product, it's important to choose collagen from a reputable source. Look for collagen that comes from grass-fed, pasture-raised animal, or from wild-caught fish. The collagen should not have any added sugars, chemical additives, artificial flavors or dyes, or additional fillers or additives like carrageenan or magnesium stearate. Ideally, you can opt for a brand that is transparent about their processes and sourcing. Also, look for collagen that is tested for purity and certified by a third-party quality-testing company such as NSF International or United States Pharmacopeia (USP).

COLLAGEN-BUYING CHECKLIST

WHAT TO LOOK FOR:

Seek out hydrolyzed collagen (also known as collagen peptides or collagen hydrolysate) or gelatin that is:

- From animals that were grass-fed, pasture raised, or wild-caught
- Tested for purity, which means the product contains the amount of the ingredient advertised on the label and isn't contaminated with dangerous substances, such heavy metals
- From a company that offers transparency about its processes and sourcing
- Third-party quality-tested by NSF International or United States Pharmacopeia (USP)

WHAT TO AVOID:

- Added sugars
- Additives
- Artificial flavors
- Artificial preservatives
- Artificial sweeteners

How Much Collagen Should I Take?

Research shows that most individuals should consume 2.5–10 grams of collagen daily. Most manufacturers recommend a serving size of about 10–20 grams of collagen peptides. Most brands include a 10-gram scoop with their products, so a serving size is typically two scoops.

When it comes to collagen (and all supplements), remember that more isn't always better. If you're eating a whole-food diet and are in good health, one scoop (which equals about two tablespoons) is a good starting point. If you're sick, stressed, recovering from childbirth, have higher-than-average protein needs, have a leaky gut or celiac disease, or have recently undergone surgery, you may want to increase your daily intake to two scoops. If you're unsure about where to start, a registered dietitian or another qualified healthcare provider can help you determine the amount that's appropriate for you.

How Long Will It Take to See Results?

Many of the clinical trials indicate that results will appear within four weeks. However, every individual is different. It's recommended to take collagen supplements indefinitely, because as we age the body produces less collagen each year. Supplementing with collagen isn't a quick fix, but rather a lifelong tool to use for aging well.

Are There Any Side Effects of Taking Collagen Supplements?

Currently, taking collagen supplements presents very few risks. However, it's important to mention that some collagen supplements are made from common food allergens, such as fish, shellfish, or eggs. If you have an allergy to these foods, you should avoid collagen supplements made with these ingredients to prevent allergic reactions.

A very small number of people have reported that collagen supplements leave a lingering bad taste in the mouth. Additionally, some individuals have reported that collagen has the potential to cause digestive side effects, such as feelings of fullness or heartburn.

Generally, these collagen supplements seem to be safe for most people, including children, pregnant women, and breastfeeding women. Even so, you should always check with your doctor before starting a new supplement, especially when pregnant, breastfeeding, or when giving the supplement to children.

Do I Need to Take Collagen on an Empty Stomach?

Many collagen advocates recommend taking collagen supplements on an empty stomach and claim that stomach acid will break down the collagen protein before it has a chance to be absorbed by the small intestine. This is a myth. Your stomach will release stomach acid and begin the digestion process as soon as any food makes its way into the stomach. Collagen isn't an exception.

Thus far, no studies have emphasized the need to take a collagen supplement on an empty stomach to reap its benefits. Gelatin may be one exception because of its ability to absorb water and coat the lining of the small intestine. If you need extra gut healing or suffer from leaky gut or other gut issues, you may find taking gelatin on an empty stomach beneficial.

Can Collagen Replace My Protein Powder?

Collagen supplements can be a good replacement for your traditional protein powder if you are eating a well-balanced diet and getting other sources of protein. If you are on a plant-based diet and do not consume much or any meat, I do not recommend relying on collagen supplements as your main source of protein, since collagen is missing essential amino acids your body needs. When collagen is paired with other protein from a plant-based or animal protein source consumed throughout the day, you are more likely to get all the amino acids your body needs.

Can I Take Collagen while Pregnant or Nursing?

Collagen is a natural form of protein that comes from animals, so it's safe to take while pregnant or breastfeeding. Taking collagen supplements while pregnant or postpartum actually offers many additional benefits. For example, protein needs increase during pregnancy. The average protein goal for most pregnant women is 70–100 grams per day. Taking collagen supplements is an easy way to boost the protein levels of nearly any food or drink. Add it to smoothies, energy bites, or raspberry leaf tea.

Collagen supplements may also help to keep bones strong throughout the pregnancy and postpartum period. During pregnancy and breastfeeding, women are at risk of increased bone loss, which reduces their bone mineral density. Research shows that collagen peptides can help support bone health by stimulating bone-forming cells and optimizing calcium absorption.

Throughout their pregnancy and postpartum period, many women experience hormonal and micronutrient shifts that cause dry skin or hair loss. This can last a year or more after the birth. Collagen supplements have been found to help with the strength and moisture content of skin and hair; therefore, they have the potential to help with these issues. They can also help with skin elasticity and hydration and can improve the appearance of wrinkles. Minimizing collagen breakdown and keeping up hydration and elasticity is thought to help reduce the chances of stretch marks.

Finally, collagen supplements have been shown to accelerate wound healing. Going through labor and birth takes quite a toll on a woman's body. During birth, collagen and elastin break down rapidly. Taking collagen can assist in the rebuilding of tissue, helping the pelvic floor, abdominal muscles, and uterus to heal. During the postpartum period, collagen supplements can be part of a healthy, balanced diet that includes other high-quality protein sources to support optimal recovery.

It's important to note that few relevant studies have been conducted on pregnant or breastfeeding women; ethics protocols prevent scientists from conducting direct research with them. If you are interested in adding collagen while pregnant or breastfeeding, make sure you read labels and that your supplement doesn't contain other ingredients or fillers you may want to avoid during this time. Just to be on the safe side, it is best to talk with your doctor about supplements before taking any at this special time in your life.

The Bottom Line: Should I Take Collagen Supplements?

Of course, that decision is up to you! Hopefully your eyes have been opened to all the benefits of collagen supplements. We've only scratched the surface of their amazing benefits, from minimizing the appearance of fine lines and wrinkles to improving joint health and digestion. Although collagen research is still in its infancy and collagen may not be the "fountain of youth" that turns back the clock ten or twenty years, the research looks promising. So why not add collagen to your diet? You may be pleasantly surprised by how your body responds. Smoother skin, fuller hair, less joint pain, quicker muscle recovery, and improved digestive health are all in the cards.

I also encourage you to consider your diet and lifestyle as a whole and to minimize the factors that damage existing collagen. Reducing your sugar intake, quitting smoking, wearing sunscreen, and incorporating stress-reducing practices like yoga and meditation can help slow down the aging process. Focusing on a balanced diet that limits red meat and emphasizes fruits, vegetables, legumes, whole grains, and healthy fats helps ensure that you are preserving the collagen in your body and reducing your risk of heart disease and other chronic conditions. Furthermore, many plant-based foods offer important nutrients and plant extracts that support collagen production. Taking into consideration your diet and lifestyle as a whole is the only way to have an upper hand in the aging process and to optimize your health. When it comes to collagen supplements, think of them as just another tool to help you maintain optimal health.

CREATING A COLLAGEN RITUAL

Do you have rituals in place? Perhaps you have a morning routine that includes journaling, meditation, or brewing a fresh pot of coffee. Not a morning person? Maybe your rituals take place in the evening. This may include winding down with a hot bath, yoga, or a regular skin-care routine.

Even if none of these rituals resonate with you, it's important to have practices that set the tone for the day. This is where collagen can fit in. I encourage you to start thinking of collagen use as a ritual. It's something you can incorporate daily to benefit your body and optimize your health.

When you begin doing so, for example by taking ten extra minutes to sit in solitude and sip a warm beverage, it can drastically affect how you feel.

Creating rituals throughout your day and incorporating wellness practices like taking collagen are acts of self-care. These little things can make a huge difference by setting the tone for the day, helping you unwind in the evening, or giving you that refresh you need when you feel like you've hit a wall.

Incorporating collagen supplements into a daily ritual couldn't be simpler. If you already have rituals in place, taking a collagen supplement, adding collagen peptides to your morning coffee, or making a collagen-rich meal is an easy addition. If you don't have a ritual in place, I highly encourage you to create one.

Start by examining what a typical day looks like for you. It may be helpful to break it down by morning, afternoon, and evening. After you've identified your typical day, think about how you can add one thing to optimize your morning, afternoon, or evening. It could be as simple as taking collagen supplements. Maybe you've realized that to feel your best, you need to wake up ten minutes earlier to make yourself breakfast. Maybe you need to take a midday walk or drink a glass of water to help you feel refreshed. If you need help winding down at night, maybe you should try stretching or gentle yoga before bed.

By shifting your time and incorporating daily rituals, you create this sacred space to set your mind to a positive state. Collagen can be one of your rituals. Fitting it into your daily routine or creating a new routine altogether is an easy way to reap the benefits of collagen while creating a more vibrant life.

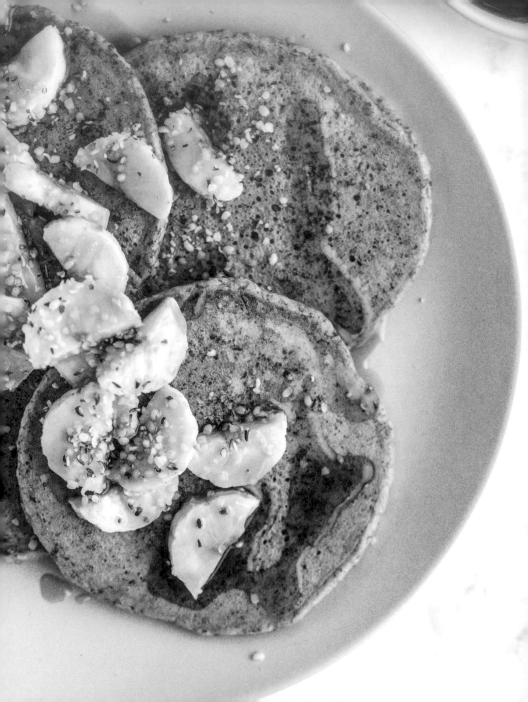

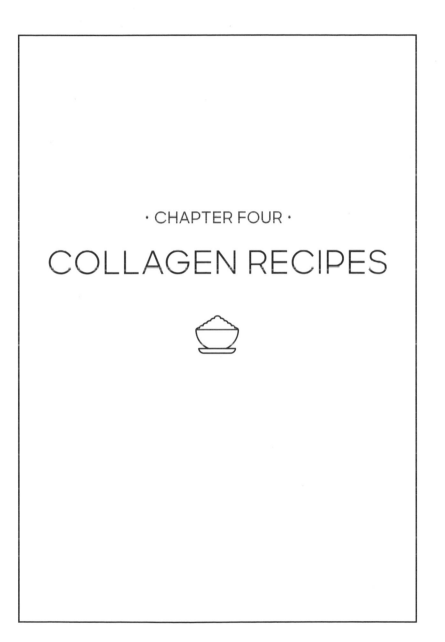

· CHAPTER FOUR ·

COLLAGEN RECIPES

Even if you regularly eat animal proteins or consider them an occasional part of your diet, you might not be eating the collagen-rich parts of food. These recipes solve this problem. Incorporating collagen peptides and the occasional helping of bone broth is an easy way to enrich your everyday recipes with the benefits of collagen and increase their protein content. Collagen peptides are tasteless and magically dissolve into almost anything. This means you can easily consume 20 grams of collagen daily by adding it to your favorite foods. You'll see just how easy it is to add collagen powder to smoothies, lattes, pancakes, soups, and sweet treats like cookies, brownies, and ice cream. All the recipes in this book are considered nutrient dense. They focus on variety and abundance, using antioxidant-rich, plant-based foods like fruits, veggies, whole grains, legumes, nuts, and seeds. They are also all dairy free and free of refined sugars.

For the recipes in this book, we will be using collagen peptides in powdered form. The recipes highlight the versatility of collagen peptides and, on occasion, bone broth. Collagen peptides are the most versatile, since they can be added to just about anything! From water to coffees, smoothies, soups, salad dressings, and baked goods, the possibilities are endless.

You may be wondering why this book focuses on recipes centered on plants if collagen is found only in animal products. There are a few reasons, but the main one comes from the research on the benefits of a mostly plant-based diet. Many studies have shown that reducing meat intake has a health-protective effect. These studies show that people who eat red meat are at an increased risk of death from heart disease, stroke, diabetes, or cancer. The more processed meats, such as salami, hot dogs, and sausages, also increase the risk of death from these diseases. But meat consumption is not the only factor in the relationship between diet and disease. Diets low in nuts, seeds, seafood, fruits, and vegetables also increase the risk of death. This is why a mostly plant-based diet, rooted in whole foods, is recognized for its role in longevity and disease prevention.

A mostly plant-based diet is based on the following principles:

- Eat mostly fruits, vegetables, legumes, and whole grains.
- Focus on plant-based protein instead of animal protein.
- View meat and other animal products as a condiment rather than the main dish.
- Eat the foods in their least processed, most natural form.
- Limit added sugar and sweets.

The foundation of my approach to nutrition focuses on a mostly plant-based diet. This means the majority of what you eat comes from plant foods. From there, you have the flexibility to choose what types of animal-based products you incorporate into your diet, if any! I have clients who eat a solely plant-based diet but choose to incorporate collagen supplements. I have others who choose to consume only eggs and fish in the realm of animal protein, while others enjoy it all. The reality is that when you have a predominantly plant-based diet, you can be flexible with the foods you choose to complement your eating style as long as they make you feel your best.

VANILLA CHAI LATTE (page 70)

COZY DRINKS
& SMOOTHIES

This section includes warm beverages, elixirs, lattes, and smoothies. The cozy drinks make it easy to incorporate collagen into your routine as a daily ritual. Taking the time to make one of these recipes is an act of self-care. Whether you're starting the day with MCT Collagen Coffee (page 72) or winding down with the Golden Turmeric Latte (page 64), taking the time to slow down and sip will do wonders for both your body and your mind.

The collagen-packed smoothie recipes were created with a specific formula in mind. Each smoothie balances protein, healthy fat, fiber, and a veggie to help keep your blood sugar stable and keep you feeling satisfied for more than an hour or two. These smoothies are the answer when you're short on time or looking for a nutrient-packed meal or snack.

GOLDEN TURMERIC LATTE

SERVES 1

This caffeine-free latte gets its vibrant golden hue from turmeric. Turmeric is an ancient spice known for its healing properties and numerous health benefits. When you mix it with creamy cashew milk and warm spices, you get a healing drink that can help reduce inflammation and stress—and even help you sleep.

INGREDIENTS

1 cup cashew milk

¼ cup filtered water

2 tablespoons collagen peptides

½ teaspoon ground turmeric

¼ teaspoon ground cinnamon

⅛ teaspoon ground ginger

A few cracks fresh-ground black pepper

DIRECTIONS

• Warm the cashew milk and water in a small saucepan over medium heat until the mixture begins to simmer. Add the warm milk and the rest of the ingredients to a blender.

• Slowly bring the speed of the blender up to high and blend until the latte is frothy and smooth. Pour the golden milk latte into your favorite mug and enjoy immediately.

NUTRITION SPOTLIGHT: Turmeric is a yellow, commonly used in curry. It has been used in traditional Indian medicine for centuries. It's a powerful antioxidant that contains the compound curcumin, which is known for its anti-inflammatory properties. Turmeric has been shown to reduce inflammation and support joint health and brain health. If its nutritional potential is to be maximized, turmeric needs to be consumed with healthy fats and black pepper. So don't skip any ingredients!

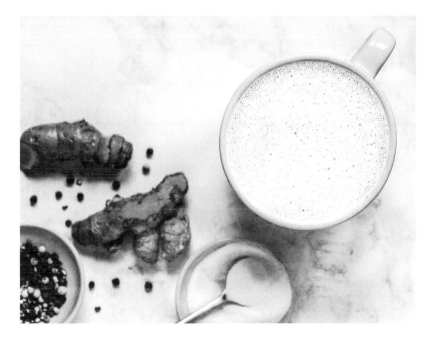

REISHI HOT CACAO

SERVES 1

A high-vibe twist on classic hot chocolate, this reishi hot cacao is made with ingredients that have amazing health benefits. Reishi mushroom has been used for centuries in ancient Chinese medicine for its healing properties and nutritional value. You can find reishi powder and other types of medicinal mushrooms like chaga, cordyceps, lion's mane, and maitake at most health food stores.

Like reishi mushroom, cacao powder has numerous health benefits. Cacao powder is less refined and therefore has a nutrition profile that is slightly superior to that of traditional cocoa powder. Cacao powder is rich in iron, calcium, magnesium, and antioxidants like theobromine. When it's blended with warm cashew milk and dates, you get a luscious, cozy drink that can be enjoyed whenever you need a chocolate fix.

INGREDIENTS

1 cup cashew milk

2 tablespoons collagen peptides

2 Medjool dates, pitted

1 tablespoon cacao powder

½ teaspoon reishi mushroom powder

DIRECTIONS

• Warm the cashew milk in a small saucepan over medium heat until it begins to simmer. Add the warm milk and the rest of the ingredients to a blender.

• Slowly bring the blender's speed up to high and blend until the hot cacao is frothy and smooth. Pour the reishi hot cacao into your favorite mug and enjoy immediately.

NUTRITION SPOTLIGHT: Medicinal mushrooms like reishi have so many benefits thanks to their nutrients and antioxidants. They are a type of adaptogen, which means they have the ability to help the body return to balance. Most medicinal mushrooms are good sources of B vitamins, zinc, choline, manganese, vitamin D, and copper, and they contain the antioxidants beta-glucan and triterpene. These antioxidants give reishi mushrooms the ability to support immune function, lower blood pressure, improve memory and cognitive function, and reduce stress and systemic inflammation.

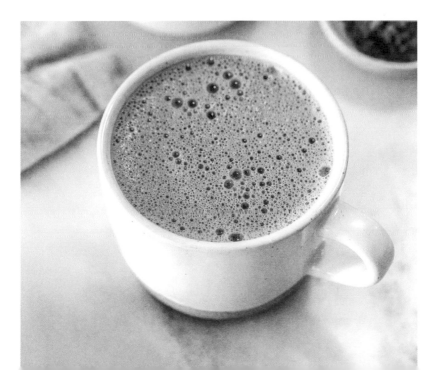

MATCHA COLLAGEN LATTE

SERVES 1

If you're looking for steady, balanced energy without the crash, matcha is for you! Matcha green tea is high in antioxidants, amino acids, and chlorophyll. L-theanine is the most prominent amino acid in matcha and is known for its relaxation effects. When paired with the small amount of natural caffeine found in the matcha leaves, it offers steady energy and focus without the traditional caffeine jitters and crash. This recipe combines high-quality matcha green tea leaves with ultra-creamy oat milk for a simple but delicious matcha latte. High-quality matcha green tea is a bright, vibrant green. This is usually classified as ceremonial-grade matcha. Avoid purchasing matcha that is dull and slightly yellow or gray.

INGREDIENTS

1 cup oat milk

¼ cup filtered water

2 tablespoons collagen peptides

1 teaspoon high-quality matcha

½ teaspoon honey, or more to taste (optional)

DIRECTIONS

• Warm the oat milk and water in a small saucepan over medium heat until the mixture begins to simmer. Add the warm milk and the rest of the ingredients to a blender. If you're new to matcha or prefer a little sweetness in your tea, you can add the ½ teaspoon of honey or more to taste.

• Slowly bring the blender's speed up to high and blend until the latte is frothy and smooth. Pour the matcha latte into your favorite mug and enjoy immediately.

NUTRITION SPOTLIGHT: Matcha differs from other green teas in that the tea leaves are ground into an extremely fine powder and consumed. Since you're consuming the entire leaf, you're getting more nutrients, antioxidants, and caffeine than if you drank typical green tea. Numerous studies have shown that matcha can help protect the liver, boost brain function, promote heart health, and even aid in weight loss.

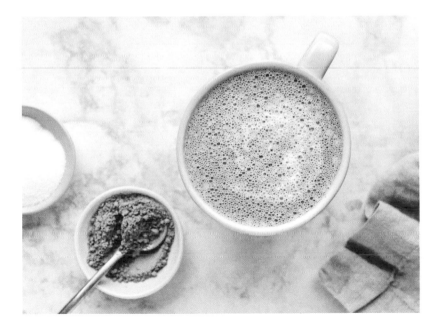

VANILLA CHAI LATTE

SERVES 1

Chai is a blend of black tea and warming spices like cinnamon, ginger, cloves, and cardamom. These spices and the black tea all have unique health benefits that are mostly related to their antioxidant properties. This vanilla chai latte is a sweet, aromatic drink that feels like a hug in a mug. Prepared chai is blended with collagen peptides, tahini, a Medjool date, and vanilla to make this unique, complex-tasting latte. Instead of using milk to add creaminess, this recipe blends tahini with the tea. Take note of this quick kitchen hack! Blending any nut or seed butter with water gives you a creamy nut or seed milk.

INGREDIENTS

2 masala chai tea bags

1½ cups filtered water

2 tablespoons collagen peptides

1 tablespoon tahini

1 Medjool date, pitted

½ teaspoon vanilla extract

DIRECTIONS

• Bring the water to a simmer in a kettle or in a small saucepan on the stove. Once simmering, remove from heat and pour into a mug with the tea bags. Let steep for 5 minutes.

• Add the steeped tea to a blender with the tahini, vanilla, collagen, and Medjool date. Slowly bring the blender's speed up to high and blend until the latte is frothy and smooth. Pour the vanilla chai latte back into the mug and enjoy immediately.

VANILLA COLLAGEN HEMP MILK

MAKES ABOUT 3 CUPS

Making your own nut or seed milk can seem daunting, but I promise you that making homemade hemp milk could not be easier. All you need are hemp seeds, water, and a blender. The best part about it is there's no straining required!

This vanilla hemp milk is a slightly sweet version that gets an extra protein boost from collagen peptides. It's delicious in smoothies and lattes or poured over a bowl of cereal. It also pairs well with the Chocolate Chip Collagen Cookies on page 119.

INGREDIENTS

3 cups filtered water

½ cup hemp seeds

2 tablespoons collagen peptides

1–2 Medjool dates, pitted

1 teaspoon vanilla extract

Pinch of fine sea salt

DIRECTIONS

• In a blender, combine the water, hemp seeds, collagen peptides, dates, vanilla, and sea salt. Slowly bring the blender's speed up to high and blend for 1–2 minutes, or until completely smooth. Pour into a glass jar and enjoy. The hemp milk keeps in the fridge for up to 5 days. It's normal for separation to occur, so make sure to shake well before using.

MCT COLLAGEN COFFEE

SERVES 1

Bulletproof® Coffee is all the rage. This trendy drink, created by David Asprey, was designed to help your body burn fat in a fasted state. It mixes coffee, grass-fed butter or ghee, and pure MCT oil. This combination is meant to serve as a breakfast replacement and comes with numerous benefits, including sustained energy, mental clarity, satiety, and antioxidants. Although there isn't much science to support all the claims of Bulletproof Coffee just yet, its ingredients have been shown to have many health benefits. This recipe is a spin-off of the traditional Bulletproof Coffee and makes a delicious beverage packed with healthy fat and protein.

INGREDIENTS

1½ cups hot, freshly brewed coffee

2 tablespoons collagen peptides

1 tablespoon MCT oil

½ tablespoon cacao butter or ghee

DIRECTIONS

• In a blender, add the coffee, collagen peptides, MCT oil, and cacao butter or ghee. Slowly bring the blender's speed up to high and blend until coffee is frothy and smooth. Pour the coffee into your favorite mug and enjoy immediately.

NUTRITION SPOTLIGHT: MCT oil is a unique fat made up of medium-chain triglycerides (MCTs). This type of fatty acid is metabolized differently than the long-chain triglycerides found in most other fat sources. MCTs are rapidly broken down and easily absorbed by the body to use as instant energy rather than stored fat.

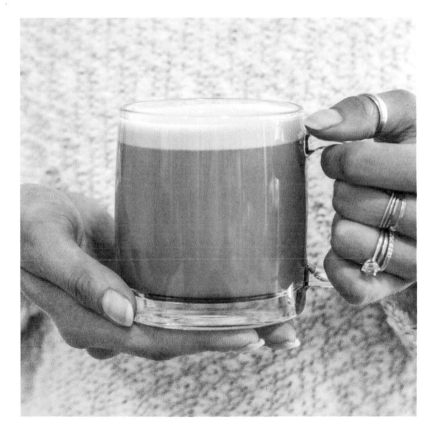

NUTRITION SPOTLIGHT: Cinnamon is a sweet spice with numerous health benefits. Ceylon cinnamon is the type of cinnamon with the most antioxidants and the unique ability to help stabilize blood sugar and keep it from spiking by imitating the effects of insulin and increasing the body's ability to transport glucose to the cells. These effects have been shown to be beneficial for someone who is eating a meal that includes carbohydrates.

BALANCED BLUEBERRY SMOOTHIE

SERVES 1

This blueberry smoothie is low in sugar and has protein, healthy fat, and fiber—a combination that is key for blood sugar balance. Stabilizing your blood sugar helps provide energy without a crash by keeping you feeling full and suppressing your hunger hormones.

Blueberries have less sugar than most fruits, but they still provide a lot of flavor. Frozen cauliflower is used in place of bananas to keep this smoothie low in sugar and give it a thick, creamy texture. Collagen peptides, almond butter, and ground flaxseed are essential for providing the necessary protein, healthy fats, and additional fiber that give this smoothie its blood-sugar balancing properties and its name.

INGREDIENTS

1 cup almond milk

½ cup frozen riced cauliflower

½ cup frozen blueberries

Juice of one lemon
(about 2 tablespoons)

¼ cup collagen peptides

1½ tablespoons ground flaxseed

1 tablespoon almond butter

⅛ teaspoon ground cinnamon

DIRECTIONS

• In an upright blender, combine the almond milk, frozen riced cauliflower, frozen blueberries, lemon juice, collagen peptides, flaxseed and cinnamon. Slowly bring the blender's speed up to high and run until the mixture is completely smooth. Enjoy immediately.

TROPICAL GREEN SMOOTHIE

SERVES 1

You'll be sipping your way to paradise with this simple smoothie. The coconut and pineapple combo gives this smoothie a piña colada vibe—a green piña colada, that is. The spinach gives this tropical green smoothie its gorgeous hue and packs in the nutrients. Spinach is incredibly rich in nutrients, making this smoothie a good source of vitamin A, vitamin K, folate, iron, and calcium.

INGREDIENTS

1 cup light coconut milk

1 large handful of spinach

½ frozen banana

½ cup frozen pineapple

¼ avocado

¼ cup collagen peptides

¼ inch knob fresh ginger

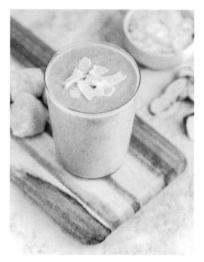

DIRECTIONS

• In an upright blender, combine the coconut milk, spinach, banana, pineapple, avocado, and collagen peptides. If using a high-speed blender, you can add the ginger in whole. Otherwise, use a microplane grater to grate in the ginger. Slowly bring the blender's speed up to high and run until mixture is completely smooth. Enjoy immediately.

SNICKERDOODLE SMOOTHIE

SERVES 1

This subtly sweet smoothie is reminiscent of a deliciously spiced snicker-doodle cookie. It's like having dessert but as a healthy, veggie-packed smoothie. Using frozen riced cauliflower in this smoothie cuts the sugar while still giving the smoothie a thick, creamy texture. The almond milk and almond butter, combined with vanilla, cinnamon, and almond extract, give it its unique cookie-inspired flavor.

INGREDIENTS

1 cup almond milk

1 cup frozen riced cauliflower

1–2 Medjool dates, pitted

1 tablespoon almond butter

1 tablespoon ground flaxseed

¼ cup collagen peptides

2 teaspoons vanilla extract

½ teaspoon almond extract (optional)

⅛ teaspoon ground cinnamon

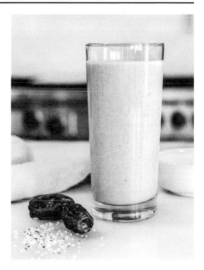

DIRECTIONS

• In an upright blender, combine the almond milk, frozen riced cauliflower, dates, almond butter, ground flaxseed, collagen peptides, vanilla, almond extract, and cinnamon. Slowly bring the blender's speed up to high and run until the mixture is completely smooth. Enjoy immediately.

CHOCOLATE COLLAGEN SMOOTHIE

SERVES 1

This sweet, creamy chocolate smoothie is the perfect way to satisfy your sweet tooth without reaching for a chocolate bar. It's packed with good-for-you ingredients but tastes like a chocolate shake. The frozen riced cauliflower and banana create a thick, creamy base without overloading the smoothie with sugar. Collagen peptides add protein without compromising taste and texture. Using full-fat almond milk rather than almond milk with only 2–4 grams of fat makes this smoothie extra creamy and even more satisfying.

INGREDIENTS

1 cup almond milk

½ cup frozen riced cauliflower

½ frozen banana

¼ cup collagen peptides

1 tablespoon cacao powder

1 tablespoon almond butter

2 teaspoons vanilla

⅛ teaspoon ground cinnamon

DIRECTIONS

• In an upright blender, combine the almond milk, frozen riced cauliflower, banana, collagen peptides, cacao powder, almond butter, vanilla, and cinnamon. Slowly bring the blender's speed up to high and run until the mixture is completely smooth. Enjoy immediately.

NUTRITION SPOTLIGHT: Cacao powder is different from traditional cocoa powder used in baking or in hot chocolate mixes. Cacao powder is less processed and richer in nutrients than cocoa powder. It's extremely high in flavonoids and polyphenols, which act as antioxidants in the body. These compounds help fight free radicals. Free radicals are atoms in the body with unpaired electrons; they cause damage in the body called oxidative stress, which shows up as inflammation, aging, and other diseases. Cacao is also a good source of magnesium, iron, zinc, potassium, phosphorus, and copper.

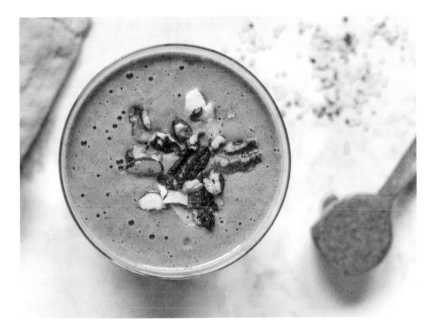

PINK PITAYA BOWL

SERVES 1

The smoothie base for this bowl gets its vibrant pink color from pitaya (also known as dragon fruit). Pitaya is a tropical fruit native to Central America. It has a mildly sweet taste that is something of a cross between a kiwi and a pear. Although there is also white pitaya, pink pitaya has grown in popularity due to its unforgettable magenta hue. Fresh pitaya can be hard to come by, but most health food stores are jumping on the pitaya trend and carry frozen pink pitaya in the freezer section.

Since this fruit is more for show than flavor, this smoothie bowl gets a flavor boost from sweet banana and fresh lemon juice. You can also add flavor by getting creative with the toppings. Coconut flakes, fresh fruit, granola, or a sprinkle of nuts or seeds are a few of my favorites.

INGREDIENTS

½ cup almond milk

1 cup frozen riced cauliflower

1 (3.5-ounce) packet frozen pink pitaya

Juice from ½ lemon (about 1 tablespoon)

½ frozen banana

¼ cup collagen peptides

DIRECTIONS

• In an upright blender, combine the almond milk, frozen riced cauliflower, pitaya, lemon, banana, and collagen peptides. Slowly bring the blender's speed up to high and run until the mixture is completely smooth. You may need to use the tamper or scrape down the sides to make sure it's fully blended. Enjoy immediately with your favorite toppings.

NUTRITION SPOTLIGHT: Pitaya or dragon fruit has white or pink flesh speckled with tiny black seeds throughout. The outer skin is either bright pink or yellow with green scales that make it look like a dragon—hence the name. Although pitaya might be known for its color, it is very nutritious. Despite being low in calories, it contains fiber, magnesium, iron, and numerous antioxidants.

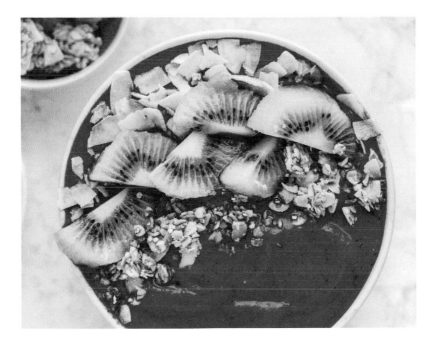

CASHEW COCONUT
COLLAGEN BITES (page 84)

SMALL BITES

This section is filled with small-bite recipes that make the perfect snack, appetizer or crowd-pleaser. There is an array of snacks that you can premake and have on hand when you need a quick midday pick-me-up, as well as dips and spreads that make for crowd-favorite appetizers or game day snacks. Sharing these collagen-packed snacks with your friends is highly encouraged. That way you can all benefit from the collagen boost!

CASHEW COCONUT COLLAGEN BITES

MAKES ABOUT 15 BITES

Healthy fats are essential for keeping blood sugar stable and helping the body absorb fat-soluble vitamins, such as vitamins A, D, E, and K, and fat-soluble antioxidants like lycopene and beta-carotene. Fats help form every cell in the body, protect organs, regulate hormones, curb cravings, and keep hair and skin strong, healthy, and glowing.

These little bites are packed with healthy fats and important nutrients from cashews, almonds, and coconuts. These cashew coconut collagen bites make the perfect afternoon pick-me-up and can be eaten as needed for a sustained source of energy.

INGREDIENTS

1 cup cashews

½ cup almonds

½ cup unsweetened coconut flakes, plus ¼ cup for rolling, if desired

1–2 pitted Medjool dates or 2–5 drops of stevia (optional)

¼ cup collagen peptides

½ cup almond or cashew butter

¼ cup coconut butter, melted and cooled (can substitute coconut oil but bites won't be as firm)

2 teaspoons vanilla extract

½ teaspoon ground cinnamon

¼ cup hemp seeds, for rolling (optional)

DIRECTIONS

• In a food processor, blend together the cashews, almonds, coconut flakes, and dates (if using), until small crumbles form.

• Add the collagen peptides, almond butter, coconut butter, cinnamon, and vanilla. Pulse until ingredients come together and start to form a dough. This will take about 15–20 pulses or about 30 seconds. Be careful not to overprocess or you'll make nut butter.

• The dough will be sticky, but that's okay! Place the mixture in the freezer for 5–10 minutes to firm up. Once it's chilled, scoop a heaping tablespoon and roll it into a ball. Repeat with the rest of the mixture. You should end up with about 15 bites. Once balls are formed, you can roll them in coconut flakes or hemp seeds, if desired. Store in an airtight container in the fridge for 2 weeks or freeze for 2 months. If storing in the freezer, let thaw for 5 minutes before eating.

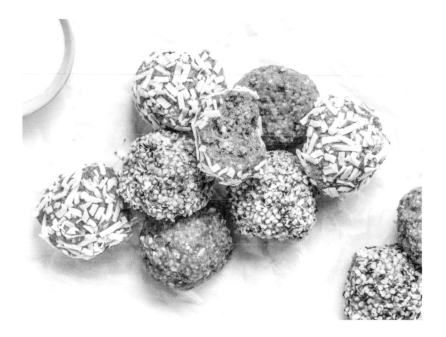

OATMEAL COOKIE COLLAGEN BITES

MAKES ABOUT 14 BITES

Soft and chewy oatmeal cookies are turned into a protein-packed, no-bake snack bite with this recipe. These will be your go-to the next time you're craving a classic oatmeal cookie but can't imagine turning on the oven. Rolled oats, almond flour, cashew butter, and dates give these protein bites a traditional oatmeal cookie vibe. When it comes to oatmeal cookie add-ins, you're either team chocolate chips or team raisins, so I'll let you decide. Either way, these oatmeal cookie collagen bites are delicious.

INGREDIENTS

1½ cups quick-cooking
    rolled oats

5 Medjool dates, pitted

¼ cup collagen peptides

¼ cup almond flour

⅓ cup cashew butter

2 teaspoons vanilla extract

Pinch of fine sea salt

2 tablespoons filtered water
    (optional)

⅓ cup raisins, chopped Bing
    cherries, or dark chocolate
    chips

DIRECTIONS

• In a food processor, blend 1 cup oats and the dates until a crumble forms.

• Add the collagen peptides, almond flour, cashew butter, vanilla, and salt. Pulse until ingredients come together and start to form a dough. This will take about 15–20 pulses or about 30 seconds. You may need to add 2 tablespoons of filtered water to help the dough stick together. Add in the additional ½ cup of oats and the chocolate chips, Bing cherries, or raisins. Pulse 10 times to distribute throughout the dough.

• Scoop a heaping tablespoon of the mixture and roll into a ball. Repeat with the rest of the mixture. You should end up with about 14 bites. Store in an airtight container in the fridge for 2 weeks or the freezer for 2 months.

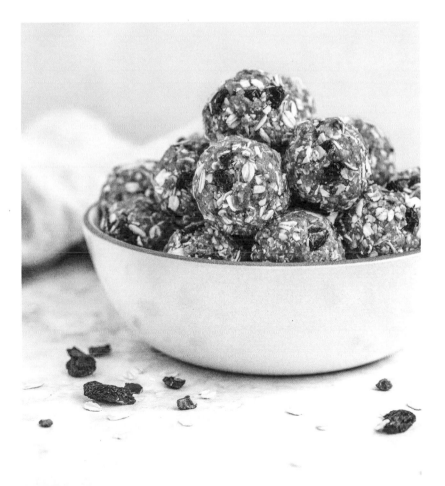

RASPBERRY CHIA SEED PUDDING PARFAIT

SERVES 4

Chia pudding is incredibly easy to make and packed with healthy omega-3s and fiber. This recipe takes my go-to vanilla collagen chia pudding and elevates it with a layer of simple raspberry compote and a handful of toppings for more flavor and texture. I purposefully kept the chia pudding unsweetened so that it can pair with sweet raspberries. Feel free to add maple syrup or another sweetener of your choice. I recommend starting with 1 teaspoon.

INGREDIENTS

For the Vanilla Chia Pudding:

½ cup chia seeds

2 cups plant-based milk of choice

⅓ cup collagen peptides

2 teaspoons vanilla extract

Pinch of cinnamon

For the Raspberry Compote:

1 cup frozen raspberries

2 teaspoons maple syrup

Juice of ½ lemon (about 1 tablespoon)

½ teaspoon vanilla extract

Optional toppings:

Greek-style yogurt, almond butter, fresh or frozen raspberries, toasted coconut, hemp seeds

DIRECTIONS

• Make the chia pudding. In a large bowl, combine the plant milk, chia seeds, collagen peptides, vanilla, and cinnamon. Stir with a whisk until well combined. (Make sure all the chia seeds are coated in milk and there are no dry chia seeds floating on top. This helps ensure they'll absorb the milk.) Cover and refrigerate for at least 30 minutes but ideally 2 hours or overnight.

• For the raspberry compote, warm the raspberries and maple syrup in a small saucepan over medium-low heat. This can also be done in the microwave by heating the raspberries and maple syrup in a microwave-safe bowl for 1 minute and 30 seconds. Smash the warm berries with the back of a wooden spoon until a syrup forms. Remove from heat and add the lemon juice and vanilla.

• To assemble, you can layer the pudding and compote between four small containers and store them in the fridge for the next few days. Otherwise, keep the chia pudding and compote in separate containers and layer them just before serving. Start by layering the raspberry compote. Top with chia seed pudding and any toppings of your choice. The chia pudding and compote keeps well in an airtight container for up to 5 days.

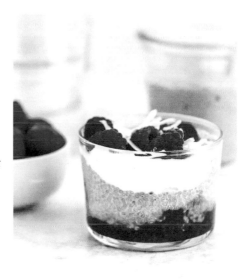

NO-CHEESE COLLAGEN QUESO

MAKES ABOUT 3½ CUPS

Rich and creamy queso without the cheese! That's right—this dairy-free queso levels up to the traditional spicy, gooey cheese dip, but it's made without any inflammatory dairy or oils. The combination of cashews and potatoes make this queso silky smooth, and the carrots give it a beautiful yellow hue. Nutritional yeast gives this queso its classic umami, cheesy flavor without any cheese. The arrowroot is optional, but it gives the queso a thick, velvety mouthfeel.

Serve the warm, gooey queso as a dip alongside organic tortilla chips. Get a little more creative and drizzle it over fajitas, tacos, burrito bowls, or steamed veggies like broccoli or cauliflower. Or toss it with some cooked noodles for an epic dairy-free mac and cheese.

INGREDIENTS

1 cup russet potato, peeled and diced

½ cup orange or yellow carrots, diced

½ cup raw cashews or sunflower seeds

3 cups vegetable stock or filtered water

½ cup nutritional yeast

¼ cup collagen peptides

Juice from ½ lemon (about 1 tablespoon)

1 teaspoon fine sea salt

½ teaspoon garlic powder

½ teaspoon smoked paprika

½ teaspoon chili powder

½ teaspoon ground cumin

¼ teaspoon cayenne pepper

1 tablespoon arrowroot powder (optional)

¼ cup pico de gallo (optional)

2 tablespoons fresh cilantro, chopped (optional)

DIRECTIONS

• Place the potatoes, carrots, cashews, and vegetable stock in a medium pot and bring to a boil. Turn the heat down slightly and let simmer until vegetables are tender and can be pierced with a fork, about 10–12 minutes.

• Add the nutritional yeast, collagen peptides, lemon juice, salt, spices, and arrowroot powder to an upright, vented blender. Add the warm potatoes, carrots, cashews, and stock. With a slightly vented lid and while holding the top with a dish towel, blend all the ingredients together. Start slowly, then blend on high for about 2 minutes. Taste, and add more salt or spices if necessary. Place hot queso in a bowl and top with pico de gallo and cilantro, if using. Serve immediately with your favorite tortilla chips. To reheat, place on the stovetop over medium heat until heated through. You may need to add more vegetable broth or water to thin the consistency.

NUTRITION SPOTLIGHT: Nutritional yeast, also known as "nooch," looks like small yellow flakes. It's often used as a vegan cheese replacement since it has a "cheesy" flavor. In addition to a unique taste, nutritional yeast has a unique nutrition profile. It's packed with protein and B vitamins. Two tablespoons of nutritional yeast has 5 grams of protein. This is quite a bit of plant-based protein packed into a small amount! Aside from using it in the queso recipe, sprinkle it on salad, grains, or pasta for an added nutrition boost!

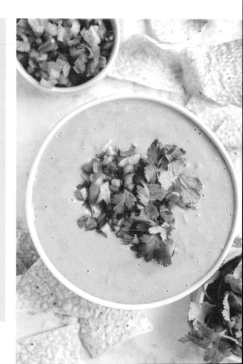

PINK COLLAGEN KETCHUP

MAKES 2 CUPS

This vibrant beet ketchup is an incredibly colorful, antioxidant-rich dip that is sure to impress. In place of tomatoes, raw red beets give the ketchup a bright pink hue. Adding collagen makes this a protein-packed condiment to pair with your favorite fries or burger.

INGREDIENTS

4 medium red beets, peeled and diced

1½ cup filtered water, divided

¼ cup collagen peptides

⅓ cup apple cider vinegar

⅓ cup coconut or date sugar

1 tablespoon Worcestershire sauce

½ teaspoon garlic powder

½ teaspoon fine sea salt

¼ teaspoon black pepper

DIRECTIONS

• Bring beets and 1 cup of water to a boil in a medium saucepan. Once boiling, turn the heat down to a simmer and cover with a lid. Cook until beets are soft and most of the liquid has evaporated, about 10 minutes. Add the beets to a blender with the ½ cup water, collagen peptides, vinegar, coconut sugar, Worcestershire sauce, garlic powder, sea salt, and pepper. Blend until smooth. The ketchup keeps well, refrigerated, for up to a week.

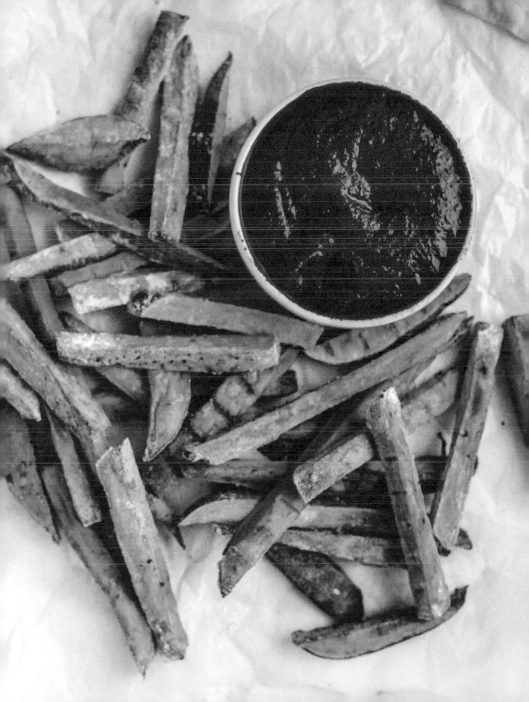

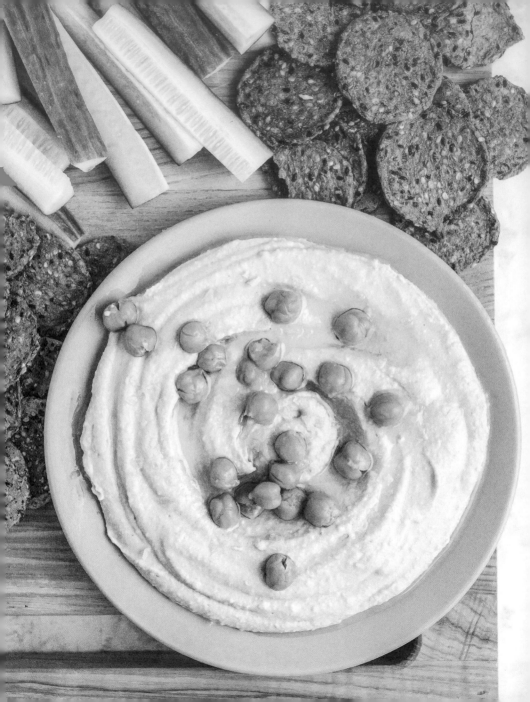

CLASSIC COLLAGEN HUMMUS

MAKES 2 CUPS

This classic hummus is thick and creamy. It's perfect for dipping, adding to salads or grain bowls, or slathering on warm flatbread. Traditional hummus starts with cooking dried beans, but that isn't ideal if you want hummus now. Canned chickpeas make this recipe come together in minutes. The nuttiness of the tahini is balanced by the brightness of the fresh lemon juice. Once you get the hang of this basic recipe, feel free to get creative. Try adding roasted red peppers, raw beets, sun-dried tomatoes, or avocado.

INGREDIENTS

2 (15-ounce) cans chickpeas, drained and rinsed

⅓ cup tahini

⅓ cup filtered water

¼ cup collagen peptides

1 lemon, juiced (about 2 tablespoons)

½ teaspoon garlic powder

1 teaspoon salt

DIRECTIONS

• Place all ingredients in a food processor and purée until smooth. Stop occasionally to scrape down the sides. This will ensure the ingredients are fully blended. The hummus can be served right away, but it's best if it's made the day before so the flavors have time to develop. Store in the fridge for up to a week.

COLLAGEN NUT AND SEED BUTTER

MAKES 2 CUPS

When it comes to nut butters, most have added sugar or oil, which is completely unnecessary. High-quality nut butters without these ingredients are out there, but they are often very expensive. It might be easier and more convenient to just pick up a jar of your favorite nut butter at the store, but I promise—making your own is well worth it.

This collagen nut and seed butter uses a delicious blend of nuts and seeds that add a variety of nutrients. This recipe is an easy way to get in your daily dose of collagen, especially if you're eating this nut and seed butter multiple times a day. Feel free to change up the combination of nuts and seeds or to use a different ratio of the suggested combination. This is a great way to use up whatever nuts or seeds you have on hand.

INGREDIENTS

4 cups any combination of nuts and seeds (for example,
    1 cup almonds, 1 cup cashews, 1 cup sunflower seeds,
    ½ cup pumpkin seeds, ½ cup Brazil nuts)

2–3 large pinches of fine sea salt

¼ cup collagen peptides

DIRECTIONS

• Roast the nuts and seeds together with the salt at 300°F for about 15–20 minutes, or until golden brown. Skip this step if using roasted, unsalted nuts. Let the nuts cool before adding to the food processor.

• Transfer the cooled, roasted nuts and seeds and salt to a food processor or high-speed blender. Run the food processor or blender on high speed for 10–20 minutes depending on the strength of your appliance. Stop and scrape down the sides a few times to ensure the ingredients are fully blended. The mixture will have a fine, powdery texture at first, but just be patient and let the food processor do its magic. The nut butter is ready when it is smooth, creamy, and runny. Taste and add more salt if needed.

• Add the collagen peptides and blend for another few seconds, until the mixture is combined. Transfer to clean glass jars. The nut and seed butter lasts for up to 2 weeks in the fridge. No separation will occur, so there's no need to stir before each use.

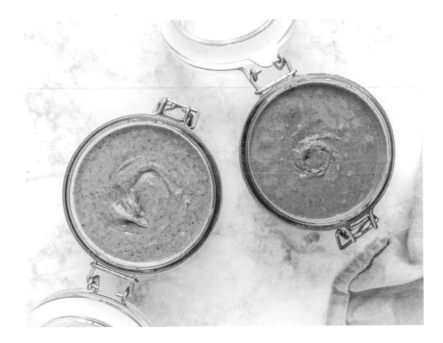

CALIFORNIA CAESAR SALAD
(page 104)

ENTREES

This section has a variety of breakfast, lunch, and dinner recipes that demonstrate just how easy it is to incorporate collagen into your favorite dishes. The goal for these recipes was to make them delicious and rich in nutrients without being overly complicated. I can confidently say that each of these recipes fits that description. Plus, many of the recipes make a large-enough batch to feed four or have leftovers for the week. This is efficiency at its finest! Whether you're feeding your family or making a dish just for yourself, you can feel confident about nourishing your body or the ones you love with these collagen-packed recipes.

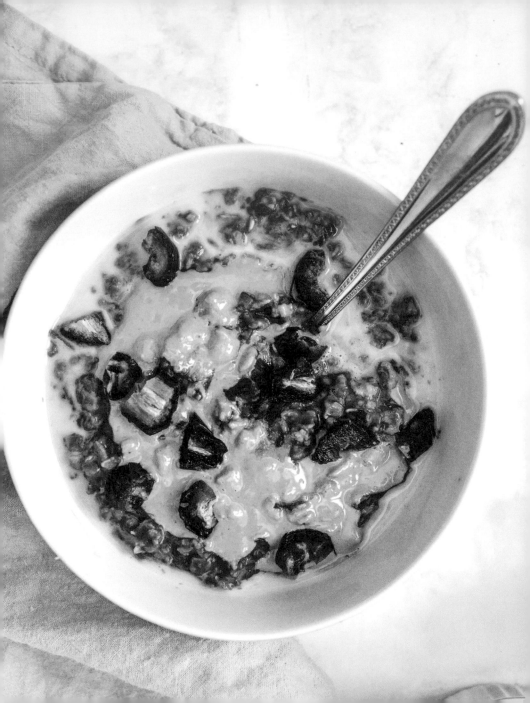

CHOCOLATE CASHEW OATMEAL BOWL

SERVES 1

This oatmeal tastes incredibly decadent for being such a nutritious breakfast. Raw cacao powder gives this oatmeal bowl its chocolaty flavor and a boost of antioxidants. The salty cashew butter and sweet Medjool dates give the bowl a peanut-butter-cup vibe. I recommend heating up your cashew butter if you want it to create that cozy-looking cashew butter pool.

INGREDIENTS

½ cup rolled oats

¾ cup almond milk

1 teaspoon vanilla extract

2 tablespoons collagen peptides

2 teaspoons cacao powder

2 teaspoons maple syrup (optional)

Toppings:

¼ cup almond milk

1½ tablespoons cashew butter

1 Medjool date, chopped

DIRECTIONS

• In a small saucepan, combine the oats, almond milk, and vanilla. Bring to a boil and let cook for 5 minutes. Add water, one tablespoon at a time, if the oatmeal starts to look dry.

• Once cooked, add in the collagen peptides, cacao powder, and maple syrup. Add more water or plant milk to thin, if necessary.

• Place in a bowl. Top with more almond milk, cashew butter, and chopped dates.

ALMOND FLOUR PANCAKES

SERVES 2

Light and fluffy almond flour pancakes (pictured on page 58) are a great way to start the day without having to worry about a mid-afternoon "pancakes crash." (You know that feeling when you need a nap after a carb-heavy breakfast? That's what I call a "pancake crash.") When you eat a stack of pancakes and don't balance it out with protein, fiber, and healthy fats, your blood sugar goes for a roller-coaster ride. After a huge spike, it comes crashing down only to leave you feeling tired, hangry, and craving more simple carbs.

This is why these almond flour pancakes are a great alternative. They're packed with protein and healthy fats to keep your blood sugar steady, with no afternoon crash. Aside from being nutritious, they're also delicious! The almond flour gives these pancakes a rich, buttery taste even though they're dairyfree. I like serving these with hemp seeds, fresh fruit, and a touch of maple syrup.

INGREDIENTS

2 large eggs

⅓ cup almond milk

1 tablespoon maple syrup

1 teaspoon vanilla extract

1 cup almond flour

¼ cup collagen peptides

½ teaspoon baking powder

¼ teaspoon cinnamon

Pinch of salt

Avocado oil spray or coconut oil

For Serving:

Sliced banana, hemp seeds, maple syrup

DIRECTIONS

• In a large bowl, whisk together the eggs, almond milk, maple syrup, and vanilla until smooth. Add in almond flour, baking powder, cinnamon, and a pinch of salt. Stir with a spoon until well combined.

• Lightly coat a large nonstick skillet with avocado oil or coconut oil and warm over medium-low heat. Spoon about 2–3 tablespoons of the batter onto the warm pan. Wait patiently until bubbles appear on top and the edges are cooked, about 5 minutes. You may need to lower the heat if you find that the pancakes are browning too quickly. Flip pancakes and cook until golden brown, about 2 minutes. Remove the cooked pancakes to a cooling rack until ready to serve. This prevents the bottom of the pancakes from getting soggy.

• Wipe skillet clean and repeat to make additional pancakes with the remaining batter.

• Serve the pancakes with sliced banana, hemp seeds, and a drizzle of maple syrup.

NUTRITION SPOTLIGHT: Almond flour is a grain-free flour alternative. It's made from finely ground blanched almonds, so it contains all the nutrients and health benefits of whole almonds. It is also significantly lower in carbohydrates than grain flours, which helps prevent the drastic blood sugar spike that can happen with other flours. Almond flour is also packed with healthy fats; minerals such as calcium, magnesium, and iron; and vitamin E for healthy skin and nails. It's important to note that almond flour is not a 1-for-1 replacement for grain flour. You often need more eggs and less liquid, so it's best to follow a recipe when using almond flour.

CALIFORNIA CAESAR SALAD

SERVES 4-6

The traditional Caesar salad gets a healthy California-style makeover. A mix of finely chopped romaine and kale is livened up with hemp seeds, vegan parmesan, and simple sourdough croutons. The real star of this salad is the creamy tahini Caesar dressing. Don't be daunted by the ingredient list. The collagen-infused dressing is incredibly easy to make—it all comes together in a blender.

INGREDIENTS

2 thick slices sourdough bread, cubed

1 tablespoon avocado oil spray or olive oil

3 cups romaine lettuce, chopped

3 cups lacinato kale, finely chopped

2 tablespoons vegan parmesan cheese or nutritional yeast

2 tablespoons hemp seeds

Salt and pepper, to taste

For the Dressing:

½ cup tahini

¾ cup filtered water, plus more to thin

¼ cup collagen peptides

2 tablespoons nutritional yeast

Juice of one lemon (about 2 tablespoons)

2 teaspoons Dijon mustard

2 teaspoons drained capers

½ teaspoon garlic powder

½ teaspoon coconut aminos or gluten-free tamari

½ teaspoon fine sea salt

¼ teaspoon pepper

DIRECTIONS

• Preheat the oven to 300°F. Line a baking sheet with parchment paper.

• Place the sourdough bread cubes on the lined baking sheet. Spray with avocado oil or drizzle with olive oil and toss to coat. Season with salt and pepper. Bake for 20–30 minutes, or until bread is golden brown and crunchy.

• Meanwhile, make the dressing. Combine all dressing ingredients in a blender. Blend until smooth. Taste and season with salt and pepper. Add extra water to thin to your liking.

• In a large bowl, toss together the romaine lettuce and kale. Pour on the dressing and toss. Top the salad with hemp seeds, vegan parmesan or nutritional yeast, and sourdough croutons. The dressed salad is best eaten immediately. If you're making it ahead of time, store the salad and dressing separately. The salad mix can be kept in the fridge for up to 5 days. The dressing will last for a week in an airtight container in the fridge.

NUTRITION SPOTLIGHT: Sourdough bread uses naturally occurring yeast and lactic acid bacteria that are present in flour to leaven the bread. This fermentation process gives sourdough bread its distinct tangy flavor and many of its health benefits. Sourdough bread allows for better absorption of nutrients because of its lower phytate levels. Phytates found in grains are considered antinutrients because they bind to minerals, reducing your body's ability to absorb them. Sourdough bread may also be easier to digest because it contains less gluten than traditional bread and has probiotic properties from the bacteria.

GLOW BOWL WITH TURMERIC TAHINI DRESSING

SERVES 2

Nourishing bowls are one of my absolute favorite dishes to make. Most of the time, I don't follow a recipe and just use up what I have on hand. But I always try to follow this simple formula. All my bowl meals have raw and cooked veggies, protein, and complex carbs as a balanced base. This gets topped with healthy fat in the form of a delicious sauce, avocado, nuts, or seeds. To provide an extra boost of nutrition and flavor, I like to add some type of fermented vegetable. This makes a balanced meal that is full of variety and extremely satisfying.

This glow bowl with turmeric tahini dressing is one of my favorites. The turmeric dressing is bright and creamy and has the most gorgeous golden hue. It's packed with antioxidants from the turmeric and has a boost of protein from the collagen. This recipe makes more dressing than needed for the two glow bowls. Store it in the fridge and use it as a salad dressing or as a dip for veggies throughout the week.

INGREDIENTS

1 cup cauliflower, chopped

1 cup sweet potatoes, diced

1 cup cooked quinoa

½ cup microgreens or watercress

¾ cup fermented vegetables (like purple cabbage or beets) or sauerkraut

2 tablespoons pumpkin seeds

Salt and pepper

Avocado oil spray

For the Dressing:

1 cup tahini

½ cup water, plus more to thin

¼ cup collagen peptides

Juice from 1 lemon (about
    2 tablespoons)

1-inch knob fresh turmeric root
    (or 1 teaspoon ground turmeric)

1 garlic clove, grated over a
    microplane

Salt and pepper, to taste

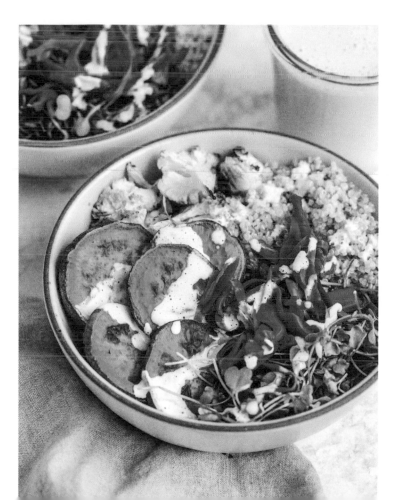

DIRECTIONS

• Preheat the oven to 400°F. Line a baking sheet with parchment paper. Place the diced cauliflower and sweet potatoes on the baking sheet. Spray with avocado oil to lightly coat. Season with salt and pepper. Place the baking sheet in the oven for 30–40 minutes, tossing the veggies halfway through.

• Meanwhile, make the dressing. Place all the dressing ingredients in a blender. Blend until completely smooth. Taste and season with salt and pepper.

• To assemble the bowls, plate the quinoa and top with the microgreens, roasted veggies, and fermented cabbage. Drizzle with the turmeric tahini dressing and top with pumpkin seeds. Place leftover dressing in an airtight container and store in the fridge for a week.

NUTRITION SPOTLIGHT: Fermentation is a process that uses microorganisms such as yeast and bacteria to preserve food. During this process, the microorganisms convert starch and sugar found in the food into alcohol or acids. The alcohol or acids act as a natural preservative. Aside from preserving foods, the benefit of fermentation is that it promotes the growth of probiotics. These beneficial bacteria have been shown to improve immune function, digestive health, heart health, and mood and to support weight loss. Some of the most common fermented foods are sauerkraut, sourdough bread, kefir, kombucha, wine, and yogurt.

VEGETABLE CHICKPEA CURRY

SERVES 4-6

This curry isn't the most traditional, but it is quick and nutritious. Most of the flavor comes from the onion and garlic caramelizing in the ghee (or coconut oil) and from the bold addition of ginger and turmeric. This curry is also packed with veggies. The recipe calls for specific vegetables, but you can use whatever you have on hand. Green beans, tomatoes, eggplant, broccoli, and potatoes will all work just fine. Serve in bowls over cooked quinoa or rice and top with cashews, fresh cilantro, or any other topping of your choice. I chose to use a combination of vegetable stock and collagen peptides to give this recipe a boost of collagen, but you can replace those two ingredients with chicken bone broth.

INGREDIENTS

½ tablespoon ghee or coconut oil

1 yellow onion, diced

2 cloves garlic, grated

1 inch fresh ginger, grated

2 teaspoons ground turmeric

½ teaspoon ground cumin

1½ teaspoons fine sea salt

1 large sweet potato, chopped into 1-inch cubes

1 medium zucchini, sliced into half-moons

3 cups cauliflower florets

1 (13.5-ounce) can light coconut milk

2 cups vegetable broth

½ cup collagen peptides

1 (15-ounce) can chickpeas, drained and rinsed

2 large handfuls fresh spinach

Juice of 1 lime (about 2 tablespoons)

For Serving:

4 cups cooked rice or quinoa

Fresh cilantro, roughly
  chopped

DIRECTIONS

• Heat the coconut oil or
ghee in a large saucepan
over medium heat. Add the
onion, garlic, ginger, turmeric,
cumin, and salt to the heated
pan. Stir and cook for a few
minutes until the onion is soft.

• Add the sweet potato
to the pan and sauté 2–3
minutes. Add a splash of
water if the spices stick to
the bottom of the pan.

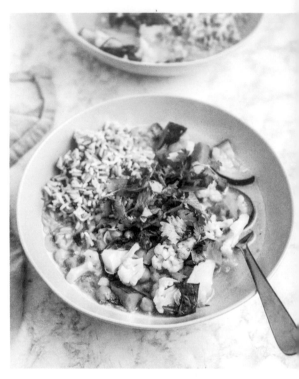

• Add the zucchini, cauliflower, and coconut milk to the pan. Then add
the vegetable broth, collagen peptides, and chickpeas. Bring to a boil,
then reduce heat to a simmer. Cook until the sweet potatoes are soft and
tender, about 15 minutes. Remove from the heat, add the spinach and
lime juice, and stir. Taste and add more salt and spices if needed.

• Serve in bowls with cooked rice or quinoa and top with fresh cilantro.
Leftover chickpea curry can be kept in an airtight container in the fridge
for up to 5 days.

GARDEN VEGGIE PESTO PASTA

SERVES 4

This recipe begs to be made with the best summer produce and fresh basil. The homemade pesto accentuates the intense flavor of the seasonal produce without being overpowering. If you've never made homemade pesto, don't be intimidated. It comes together quickly and is very forgiving. This recipe is my go-to. It's dairy free and has a boost of protein from collagen peptides. Feel free to switch up the hemp seeds for any nuts or seeds that you have on hand; cashews are a great alternative. If you're in a pinch, you can opt for store-bought pesto, but I strongly encourage giving homemade pesto at least one try.

INGREDIENTS

For the Pesto:

2 cups fresh basil

½ cup hemp seeds

1 clove garlic

Juice from 1 lemon (about 2 tablespoons)

2 tablespoons nutritional yeast or
    parmesan cheese

¼ cup collagen peptides

⅓ cup olive oil

½ teaspoon salt

¼ teaspoon black pepper

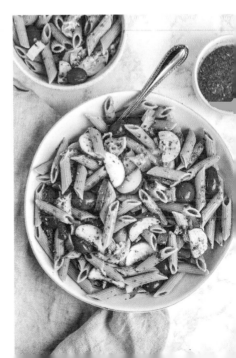

For the Pasta:

1 pound penne pasta of choice
(I recommend chickpea or
gluten-free brown rice pasta)

1 zucchini, sliced into half-moon
shapes

1 yellow squash, sliced into half-
moon shapes

½ small onion, diced

1 red or orange bell pepper, diced

1 cup cherry tomatoes

1 tablespoon olive oil

1 teaspoon salt

½ teaspoon ground pepper

DIRECTIONS

• To prepare the pesto, add all the pesto ingredients to a food processor
and blend until smooth. Taste and adjust seasoning with salt and pepper
if needed.

• Cook pasta according to package directions. Drain the pasta and
reserve ½ cup of the pasta water.

• While the pasta is cooking, heat olive oil in a large nonstick pan over
medium heat. Add all the chopped veggies to the pan and cook on
medium-high heat for 5–6 minutes, or until cherry tomatoes start to burst
and veggies are tender. Season with salt and pepper. Add the cooked pasta
to the pan with the veggies, pesto, and ¼ cup of the reserved pasta water.
Toss to coat. Add more pasta water if needed to thin.

• To serve, top with additional nutritional yeast or parmesan cheese,
if desired. Leftover pasta lasts for up to 5 days in the fridge. Store any
leftover pesto in an airtight container for up to a week.

PUMPKIN CHILI

SERVES 6

I can't wait to make chili when the weather gets colder. This pumpkin chili is meatless but still hearty and filling. The variety of beans and sautéed mushrooms gives the chili a meaty texture, and the mushrooms provide a subtle depth of flavor. The base of fire-roasted tomatoes and a whole can of pumpkin provides a heavy dose of antioxidants, vitamin C, and vitamin A.

I recommend blending half the chili and then adding it back to the pot for a thicker, less chunky chili, but it's completely optional. In place of bone broth, you can use vegetable stock and ½ cup collagen peptides.

INGREDIENTS

1 tablespoon olive oil

1 small yellow onion, chopped

1 poblano pepper, seeded and diced, or 2 ounces canned green chiles

1 cup crimini mushrooms, finely chopped

3 cloves garlic, minced or grated

2 tablespoons chili powder

2 teaspoons ground cumin

1 teaspoon fine sea salt, plus more to taste

¼ teaspoon cayenne pepper (optional)

1 (28-ounce) can crushed fire-roasted tomatoes

1 (15-ounce) can pumpkin purée

1 (15-ounce) can black beans, drained and rinsed

1 (15-ounce) can kidney or pinto beans, drained and rinsed

4 cups bone broth

Optional Toppings: Pumpkin seeds, cilantro, plain Greek-style yogurt, nutritional yeast, or shredded cheese

DIRECTIONS

• Heat a large pot over medium-high heat. Add the olive oil, onions, chili peppers, mushrooms, and 1 teaspoon of salt. Cook until the onions are translucent and the mushrooms have softened, 5–7 minutes. Then add the garlic and spices and mix to coat evenly. Cook for another 2 minutes.

• Add tomatoes, pumpkin, beans, and broth. (If using vegetable stock, add the collagen peptides at this time.) Bring mixture to a boil, then let it simmer for 20–30 minutes, or until the chili has reduced and thickened to your liking. The longer it simmers, the thicker it will get. Taste and season with more salt, if necessary.

• Use an immersion blender to blend half of it for a less chunky texture. You can also transfer half the chili to an upright, vented blender. Hold the top with a towel and blend. Then pour it back into the pot.

• Serve with pumpkin seeds, cilantro, or any of your favorite toppings. Leftovers can be stored in an airtight container in the fridge for up to 5 days.

NUTRITION SPOTLIGHT: Pumpkin is a winter squash that is packed with nutrients. It's an excellent source of vitamin K, vitamin C, and potassium and a good source of vitamin E, iron, and folate. Beta-carotene is the main antioxidant found in pumpkin; it gets converted to vitamin A in the body. Vitamin A is essential for proper immune function and healthy vision. Pumpkin is also an excellent source of fiber. One cup of pumpkin purée contains 7 grams of fiber!

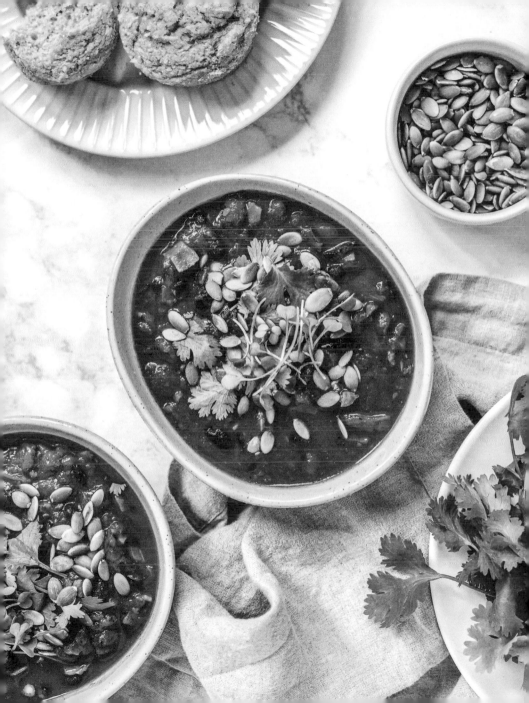

COOKIE DOUGH
FREEZER FUDGE (page 126)

SWEET TREATS

These sweet treats are made with wholesome ingredients and boosted with collagen. In place of the white cane sugar used in traditional recipes, coconut sugar, maple syrup, or dates are used to sweeten these desserts naturally. These sweeteners have a lower glycemic index, meaning they won't spike your blood sugar as high as white cane sugar does. They also provide more flavor and a slight boost of various nutrients. These collagen sweet treats are going to be your go-to recipes for elevated treats!

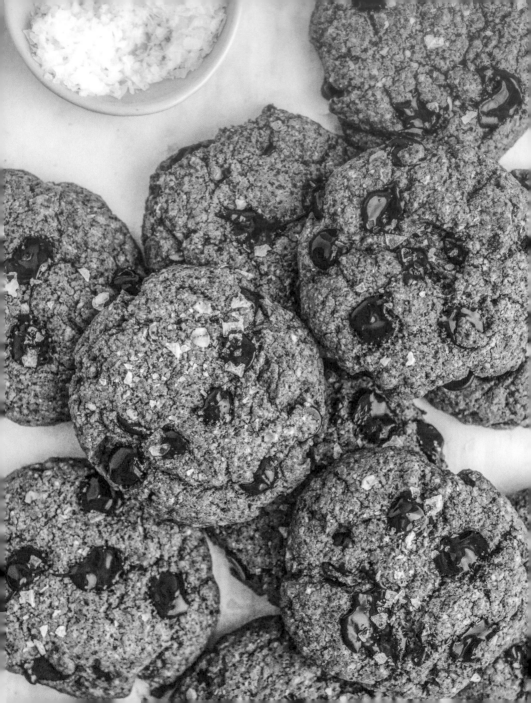

CHOCOLATE CHIP COLLAGEN COOKIES

MAKES 8-10 COOKIES

There's nothing better than biting into a warm, gooey chocolate chip cookie fresh out of the oven. It's still slightly doughy with puddles of melted chocolate, and the only way to wash it down is with a tall glass of almond milk.

These chocolate chip cookies are a wholesome version of the classic, but no less delicious. They require only ten ingredients, and chances are you already have them in your pantry. This means you have the perfect excuse to whip up a batch of these chocolate chip cookies on a whim—no special occasion required.

INGREDIENTS

⅔ cup coconut sugar

½ cup collagen peptides

1 teaspoon baking soda

½ teaspoon fine sea salt

⅓ cup dark chocolate chips

2 large eggs

1 cup unsalted creamy almond butter

2 teaspoons vanilla extract

½ cup quick-cooking rolled oats

½ cup almond flour

DIRECTIONS

• Preheat the oven to 375°F. Line a baking sheet with parchment paper.

• In a large bowl, beat the eggs with a wire whisk. Add in the almond butter and vanilla and mix with a spoon until combined. Stir in the oats, almond flour, coconut sugar, collagen peptides, baking soda, and salt until smooth. The dough will be thick. Stir in the chocolate chips. You may find it's easiest to do this using your hand.

• Scoop 2–3 tablespoons of the dough into a ball; drop it onto the prepared baking sheet. Continue until dough is used up. Gently press down on the tops of the balls to flatten slightly. Bake for 10–15 minutes, or until edges turn golden brown.

• Remove the cookies from the oven and let them cool on the pan for 10 minutes before transferring them to a wire rack to cool completely. Store cookies in an airtight container on the counter or in the fridge for 2–3 days.

NUTRITION SPOTLIGHT: Coconut sugar comes from the sap of the coconut palm tree, which is extracted, boiled, and dehydrated. Coconut sugar is caramel-colored and adds a delicious depth of flavor to baked goods. The main difference between cane sugar and coconut sugar is that coconut sugar is less refined, contains less fructose, and has more antioxidants and minerals, such as iron, zinc, calcium, and potassium. However, these nutrients are found in relatively small amounts compared to the coconut sugar content in a recipe.

FUDGY TAHINI BROWNIES

SERVES 16

These tahini brownies have all the characteristics of your favorite chewy, fudgy brownies without any of the traditional ingredients. Yes, that's right! No butter, oil, flour, or eggs. I promise you they're delicious. The tahini brings a depth of nuttiness that complements the rich, dark-chocolate flavor. It's wildly addicting, but in the best way possible!

For best results, make sure your tahini is very runny. I like Trader Joe's®, Seed + Mill, or Soom® tahini. You can also substitute another nut or seed butter—just make sure it's smooth and runny. Look for nut and seed butter with no added sugar or oils; the only ingredients should be nuts and seeds, with a little salt.

INGREDIENTS

2 eggs or 2 tablespoons ground flaxseed
  or chia seed + ⅓ cup water

1 cup tahini

½ cup coconut sugar

½ cup almond flour

½ cup collagen peptides

6 tablespoons cacao powder

2 tablespoons almond milk

½ teaspoon baking soda

¼ teaspoon fine sea salt

⅓ cup dark chocolate chips or cacao nibs

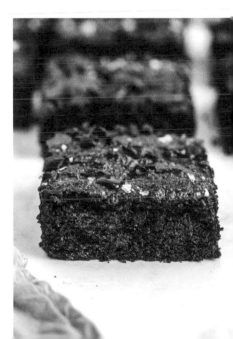

Optional Toppings:

2 tablespoons cacao nibs or more chocolate chips

Flaky sea salt

DIRECTIONS

• Preheat the oven to 350°F. Line an 8×8–inch baking pan with parchment paper. If using, make the flaxseed or chia seed egg by combining the ground flax or chia seeds with water. Let the mixture sit for 5–10 minutes until a gel forms.

• In a medium bowl, beat together the eggs with a wire whisk. Add in the tahini and coconut sugar and mix together. Add in the almond flour, collagen peptides, cacao powder, almond milk, baking soda, and sea salt, and mix well. The dough will be thick and slightly sticky. Once combined, add the chocolate chips and mix until evenly distributed. Pour the batter into the lined baking pan and smooth the top with a spatula. Sprinkle the cacao nibs or chocolate chips on top and gently press them into the batter. Finish with sea salt, if using.

• Place the pan in the oven and bake for 24–26 minutes. The edge of the brownies should be slightly crisp. You can test with a toothpick to see if they're done. A toothpick inserted into the center of the brownies should come out clean. If you want fudgy brownies, be careful not to overbake.

• Let cool for at least 15 minutes before cutting. Store leftover brownies in an airtight container in the fridge for up to 5 days.

BANANA NICE CREAM (TWO WAYS)

SERVES 2

If you're not familiar with "nice cream," you're in for a treat! It's made with frozen bananas that are blended to create the most magical soft-serve. It's ridiculously impressive how smooth and creamy frozen banana gets.

It's worth mentioning that this isn't a frozen dessert that stores well. It's best eaten immediately or after chilling for 30 minutes to 1 hour in the freezer. Any longer will require you to reblend the mixture to make it creamy again.

INGREDIENTS

Classic Vanilla:

6 small banana slices, frozen for at least 4 hours or overnight

⅓ cup full-fat cashew, almond, or coconut milk

¼ cup collagen peptides

1 teaspoon vanilla extract

Pinch of fine sea salt

Chocolate Peanut Butter:

6 small frozen banana slices

⅓ cup full-fat cashew, almond, or coconut milk

¼ cup collagen peptides

2 tablespoons cacao powder

2 tablespoons peanut butter

1 teaspoon vanilla extract

Pinch of fine sea salt

DIRECTIONS

For the Classic Vanilla:

• Place the frozen bananas in a food processor fitted with an S-blade or a high-powered blender. Add the almond milk or coconut milk, collagen peptides, vanilla, and sea salt. Puree or blend on high until smooth. You may need to scrape the bowl or use the tamper of the blender. For soft-serve-style nice cream, serve immediately or place in the freezer for 30 minutes to 1 hour for firmer nice cream.

For the Chocolate Peanut Butter:

• Place the frozen bananas in a food processor fitted with an S-blade or a high-powered blender. Add the almond milk or coconut milk, collagen peptides, cacao powder, vanilla, and sea salt. Puree or blend on high until smooth. You may need to scrape the bowl or use the tamper of the blender. Drizzle in the peanut butter and pulse until it is swirled throughout. For soft-serve-style nice cream, serve immediately or place in the freezer for 30 minutes to 1 hour for firmer nice cream.

> **NUTRITION SPOTLIGHT:** Bananas are a good source of potassium, vitamin B_6, vitamin C, fiber, and several antioxidants. Unripe bananas contain resistant starch. This acts as a prebiotic fiber, which feeds the good gut bacteria. These bacteria need to be fed if they are to stay alive and thrive. As bananas ripen, the starch turns into various sugars—glucose, fructose, and sucrose. Bananas also contain several antioxidants, which are responsible for many of their health benefits. These include dopamine and catechin. Catechins are a type of antioxidant flavonoid that has been linked to various health benefits, including a reduced risk of heart disease.

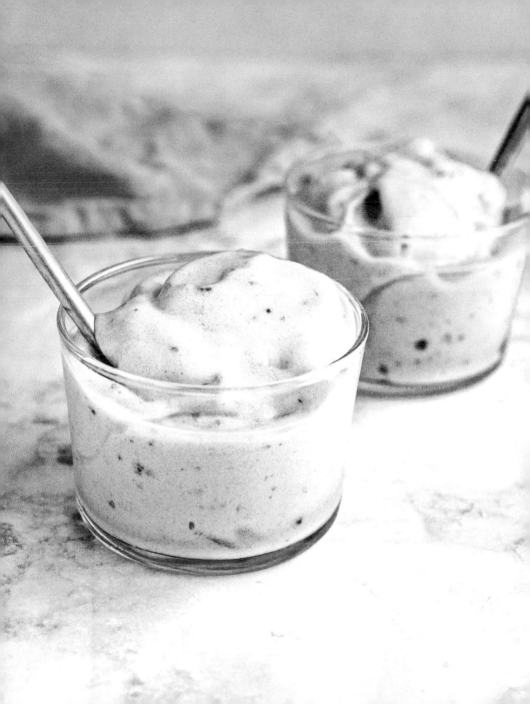

COOKIE DOUGH FREEZER FUDGE

MAKES 20 SQUARES

Whether or not they admit it, most people love eating raw cookie dough. This fudge is a more acceptable (not to mention safer!) way to satisfying your cookie dough craving. All you have to do is open your freezer.

INGREDIENTS

1 cup cashew butter

¼ cup coconut oil, melted

¼ cup collagen peptides

2 tablespoons maple syrup

2 teaspoons vanilla

½ teaspoon almond extract (optional)

¼ teaspoon salt

¼ cup dark chocolate chips, for topping

Flaky sea salt, for topping

DIRECTIONS

• Line an 8×4–inch pan with parchment paper. In a medium bowl, mix together the cashew butter, coconut oil, collagen peptides, maple syrup, vanilla, almond extract, and salt. Pour the mixture into the pan. Smooth out the top with a spatula. Sprinkle with chocolate chips, pressing down gently if necessary. Finish with a sprinkle of flaky sea salt.

• Place the pan, uncovered, on a flat surface in the freezer. Freeze for at least 30 minutes, or until the fudge is solid. Slice the fudge into about twenty 1-inch squares. Store the fudge in a freezer-safe container in the freezer for up to 3 months. Let the squares thaw for about 5 minutes before enjoying.

CHOCOLATE PEANUT BUTTER COLLAGEN CANDIES

MAKES 10 CANDIES

This recipe makes a homemade version of your favorite chocolate-covered peanut butter cups, but I'd argue it's infinitely better! Here, you're in control of the ingredients and, most importantly, the peanut butter-to-chocolate ratio. I think that those infamous peanut butter cups are seriously lacking in peanut butter. These candies, on the other hand, have a thick, slightly sweet peanut butter filling with just a light coating of your favorite dark chocolate.

Choosing high-quality ingredients makes all the difference here. I recommend using natural peanut butter that requires stirring and has only peanuts and salt as its ingredients and your favorite high-quality dark chocolate bar.

INGREDIENTS

For the Peanut Butter Filling:

½ cup salted peanut butter

1½ tablespoons maple syrup

1½ teaspoons vanilla extract

¼ cup collagen peptides

2–3 tablespoons coconut flour

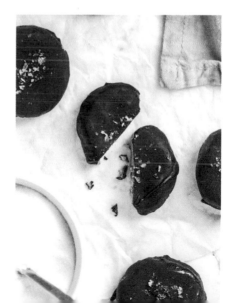

For the Chocolate Layer:

½ tablespoon coconut oil

3 ounces dark chocolate

DIRECTIONS

• To make the peanut butter cup filling, add peanut butter, maple syrup, vanilla, collagen, and 2 tablespoons of coconut flour to a medium bowl and mix until it's smooth and comes together into a thick dough. If your peanut butter is very runny, you may need to add more coconut flour. Add ½ tablespoon of coconut flour at a time until a thick dough forms. Scoop a heaping tablespoon of dough and form it into a 1½-inch thick disk. Place the disk on a small parchment-lined baking sheet or flat plate. Repeat with the rest of the dough. Once all the candies are formed, place them in the freezer for 10 minutes to chill.

• To melt the chocolate, place the dark chocolate in a microwave-safe bowl and microwave in 30-second increments until the chocolate is melted. You can also melt the chocolate in a medium saucepan over low heat, stirring frequently. Once the chocolate is melted, add the coconut oil and stir until combined.

• Remove the chilled dough from the freezer. Use two forks to dip the chilled dough in melted chocolate. Once a disk is completely coated in chocolate, let some of the excess chocolate drip from the fork before placing it back onto the parchment paper, the plate, or cooling rack. Put the chocolate-coated candies back in the freezer to harden for 15–20 minutes. Store in an airtight container in the freezer for up to 1 month or in the fridge for up to 2 weeks.

BLUEBERRY COLLAGEN CRUMBLE BARS

SERVES 12

These blueberry crumble bars are the perfect way to take advantage of fresh, juicy blueberries all summer long. The sweet, collagen-packed blueberry filling gets nestled between a lightly sweetened, crumbly dough. As the crumble bakes, the natural sugars from the fruit condense and caramelize, leaving a thick and delicious jammy filling. These bars satisfy a sweet craving and won't leave you with a sugar crash. They're perfect for a quick breakfast, snack, or healthy dessert.

If you don't have access to reasonably priced organic berries, you can use frozen blueberries without any issues. This also makes it easy to whip up these bars all year long (which I highly recommend!).

INGREDIENTS

For the Crumble:

2½ cups rolled oats, divided

½ cup almond flour

¼ cup coconut oil

¼ cup maple syrup

¼ cup applesauce or
    almond butter

1 teaspoon vanilla extract

1 teaspoon baking powder

½ teaspoon cinnamon

½ teaspoon salt

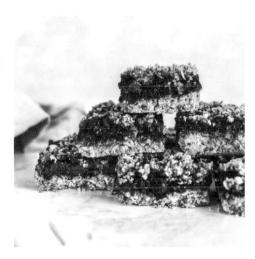

For the Filling:

3 cups frozen blueberries

3 tablespoons arrowroot powder

¼ cup collagen

Juice from 1 lemon (about 2 tablespoons)

3–4 tablespoons maple syrup (optional)

DIRECTIONS

• Preheat oven to 350°F. Line an 8×8–inch baking pan with parchment paper and set aside.

• In an upright blender or food processor, pulse 2 cups oats until ground down into a flour. Transfer to a large bowl; add the remaining ½ cup rolled oats and the rest of the crumble ingredients. Combine the ingredients until the dough begins to stick together.

• Measure a heaping ½ cup of the dough for the topping and set aside. Spread the remaining dough evenly into the prepared pan. Press firmly and flatten the dough into the bottom, sides, and corners of the pan. It may help to slightly oil or wet your fingers or spatula.

• Wipe the inside of the the food processor clean and add the blueberries. Pulse until the blueberries are broken down into small pieces. Transfer to a mixing bowl and add the remaining filling ingredients.

• Spread the filling evenly over the crumble crust. Take the remaining crumble dough and use your fingers to break it up evenly over the fruit filling. Gently push the crumble dough into the filling to set. Bake for 40–45 minutes, or until the top is golden brown and the filling is bubbling. Let the bars cool completely before slicing. Store the crumble bars in an airtight container in the fridge for up to 5 days.

PUMPKIN BREAD

SERVES 8-10

Once the weather gets cooler and the leaves start changing, it's time for pumpkin bread. There's nothing like the smell of warm spices wafting through your kitchen while this classic autumn bread bakes. This pumpkin bread gets a healthier spin by using sprouted spelt flour, collagen peptides, and maple syrup. This creates a wholesome bread that's lightly sweetened and boosted with protein and the benefits of collagen. Spelt flour is not gluten free, though it has much less gluten than traditional wheat flour. It's one of my absolute favorite flours to bake with. If you need to be gluten free, replace the spelt flour with a 1-to-1 gluten-free blend.

I tend to prefer my pumpkin bread without additions to let the soft texture shine. But feel free to mix pumpkin seeds, chopped walnuts, or chocolate chips into the batter, or sprinkle them on top before sliding into the oven.

INGREDIENTS

2 cups spelt flour or gluten-free flour blend

¼ cup collagen peptides

2 teaspoons baking powder

½ teaspoon fine sea salt

2 teaspoons ground cinnamon

½ teaspoon ground ginger

¼ teaspoon ground nutmeg

⅛ teaspoon ground cloves

1½ cups pumpkin purée

½ cup maple syrup

¼ cup almond milk

1 egg

3 tablespoons avocado or melted coconut oil

2 teaspoons vanilla

⅓ cup of extras like pumpkin seeds, chopped walnuts, chocolate chips, etc. to add to the batter or add 2–3 tablespoons on top of the loaf before baking

DIRECTIONS

• Preheat the oven to 350°F. Line an 8×4–inch loaf pan with parchment paper or grease lightly with oil.

• In a large mixing bowl, add the spelt flour, collagen peptides, baking powder, salt, and spices. Mix to combine. In a separate bowl, add the pumpkin, maple syrup, almond milk, collagen, egg, oil, and vanilla. Whisk together until completely smooth. Add the wet ingredients to the dry and mix together until just combined. Be careful not to overmix.

• Pour the batter into the loaf pan. Place in the oven for 45–50 minutes, or until a toothpick inserted into the center of the pumpkin bread comes out clean. Let sit for 10 minutes before moving to a cooling rack. Allow to fully cool before slicing. Store the pumpkin bread in the fridge for up to 5 days.

NUTRITION SPOTLIGHT: Spelt flour is an ancient strain of wheat. Even though it's not gluten free, the gluten in spelt reacts differently than the type of gluten in modern commercial wheat. It's also lower in a type of carbohydrate called fructan. Because of these unique properties, spelt can be better tolerated by some individuals who have a sensitivity to wheat or who need to be on a low FODMAP (fermentable oligo-, di-, mono-saccharides and polyols) diet for IBS (irritable bowel syndrome). It's also higher in minerals such as manganese, zinc, and copper than modern wheat. Spelt flour can easily replace traditional flour in baking recipes.

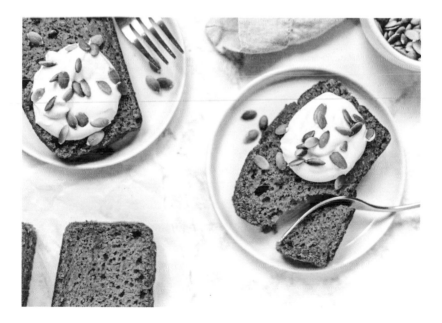

CINNAMON ROLL MUG CAKE

SERVES 1

If you've never heard of a mug cake, it's exactly what it sounds like. It's a simple cake batter that's whipped up in a mug and zapped in the microwave. The result is an incredibly moist single serving of cake that's ready in less than two minutes.

Think of this mug cake as a warm, gooey cinnamon roll without the effort. It really couldn't be easier! The simple cake batter is made with a few wholesome ingredients like oat flour, collagen peptides, maple syrup, and coconut oil. Then, a coconut sugar-cinnamon mixture is swirled throughout the batter for classic cinnamon-roll flavor. Once it's cooked, it's finished with a coconut butter glaze.

INGREDIENTS

For the Cake Batter:

¼ cup oat flour

1 tablespoon collagen peptides

½ teaspoon baking powder

A pinch of fine sea salt

¼ teaspoon cinnamon

2 tablespoons almond milk

½ tablespoon maple syrup

1 teaspoon melted coconut oil

¼ teaspoon vanilla

For the Cinnamon Swirl:

1 teaspoon melted coconut oil or ghee

2 teaspoons coconut sugar

½ teaspoon cinnamon

For the Topping:

½ tablespoon melted coconut butter

DIRECTIONS

• In a small mug or oven-safe ramekin, stir together the oat flour, collagen, baking powder, salt, and cinnamon. Add the almond milk, maple syrup, melted coconut oil, and vanilla to the dry ingredients in the mug and stir until combined.

• In a separate small bowl, make the cinnamon swirl. Add the melted coconut oil or ghee, coconut sugar, and cinnamon. Drizzle the mixture over the batter. Using a knife, gently swirl the mixture into the batter.

• Microwave on high for about 1 minute and 30 seconds (cooking time will vary with microwave wattage). Alternatively, bake at 350°F for 10–15 minutes. The mug cake is done when a toothpick inserted into the center comes out clean. Drizzle with melted coconut butter before serving. Enjoy immediately.

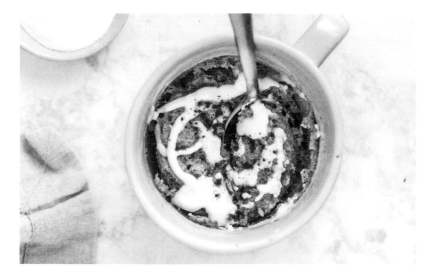

Acknowledgments

Writing this book is one of the biggest milestones of my career to date. It's always been a dream to write a book or a cookbook, but I never dreamed that it would unfold in this way. It's the perfect reminder that when you follow your dreams and put in the work, opportunities come when you least expect it.

Thank you to Ben, my husband, for always believing in me and encouraging me to do the work that lights my soul on fire. If it weren't for your support, I would not be where I am today.

Also, thank you to my family, the biggest support team I have. Mom and Dad, you have always encouraged me to dream big, pushed me to do my best, and counseled me to hang in there when times get tough. You taught me that good things come with hard work and discipline. Your words of encouragement and heartfelt affirmations always come at the perfect time. Dan, Lisa, Rose, Matt, and Sarah—thank you for constantly cheering me on. I couldn't have asked for a better family to marry into.

Thank you Nicole Fisher from Sterling Publishing for reaching out with this incredible offer. This has been the opportunity of a lifetime. Elysia Liang, you are an incredible editor. Thank you for giving this book structure and being the eye that caught my mistakes. You made this entire process a breeze.

Lastly, thank you to Year + Day for the beautiful ceramics I used to shoot the photos in this book. The modern design and matte white, pink, and gray colors created such a beautiful, cohesive style. I'm so incredibly grateful to use these quality ceramic pieces in my home.

References

Alcock, Rebekah D, Gregory C. Shaw, and Louise M. Burke. "Bone Broth Unlikely to Provide Reliable Concentrations of Collagen Precursors Compared With Supplemental Sources of Collagen Used in Collagen Research." *International Journal of Sport Nutrition and Exercise Metabolism* 29, no. 3 (May 1, 2019): 265–72. https://www.ncbi.nlm.nih.gov/pubmed/29893587.

Ambati, Ranga Rao, Siew Moi Phang, Sarada Ravi, and Ravishankar Gokare Aswathanarayana. "Astaxanthin: Sources, Extraction, Stability, Biological Activities and Its Commercial Applications—A Review." *Marine Drugs* 12, no. 1 (January 2014): 128–52. https://www.ncbi.nlm.nih.gov/pmc/articles/PMC3917265.

American Society for Dermatologic Surgery. "Cellulite." Accessed August 9, 2019. https://www.asds.net/skin-experts/skin-conditions/cellulite.

Asserin, Jérome, Elian Lati, Toshiaki Shioya, and Janne Prawitt. "The Effect of Oral Collagen Peptide Supplementation on Skin Moisture and the Dermal Collagen Network: Evidence from an Ex Vivo Model and Randomized, Placebo-Controlled Clinical Trials." *Journal of Cosmetic Dermatology* 14, no. 4 (December 2015): 291–301. https://www.ncbi.nlm.nih.gov/pubmed/26362110.

Aziz, Jazli, Hafiz Shezali, Zamri Radzi, Noor Azlin Yahya, Noor Hayaty Abu Kassim, Jan Czernuszka, and Mohammad Tariqur Rahman. "Molecular Mechanisms of Stress-Responsive Changes in Collagen and Elastin Networks in Skin." *Skin Pharmacology and Physiology* 29, no. 4 (July 20, 2016): 190–203. https://www.karger.com/Article/FullText/447017.

Bello, Alfonso E., and Steffen Oesser. "Collagen Hydrolysate for the Treatment of Osteoarthritis and Other Joint Disorders: A Review of the Literature." *Current Medical Research and Opinion* 22, no. 11 (November 2006): 2221–32. https://www.ncbi.nlm.nih.gov/pubmed/17076983.

Bertrand, Julien, Ibtissem Ghouzali, Charlène Guérin, Christine Bôle-Feysot, Mélodie Gouteux, Pierre Déchelotte, Philippe Ducrotté, and Moïse Coeffier. "Glutamine Restores Tight Junction Protein Claudin-1 Expression in Colonic Mucosa of Patients with Diarrhea-Predominant Irritable Bowel Syndrome." *Journal of Parenteral and Enteral Nutrition* 40, no. 8 (November 2016): 1170–76. https://www.ncbi.nlm.nih.gov/pubmed/25972430.

Binic, Ivana, Viktor Lazarevic, Milanka Ljubenovic, Jelena Mojsa, and Dusan Sokolovic. "Skin Ageing: Natural Weapons and Strategies." *Evidence-Based Complementary and Alternative Medicine* (2013). https://pdfs.semanticscholar.org/0a90/9f08c8d5b-3da4aaa0f3d3c46e2ed2085a5ec.pdf.

Bizot, Valérie, Enza Cestone, Angela Michelotti, and Vincenzo Nobile. "Improving Skin Hydration and Age-Related Symptoms by Oral Administration of Wheat Glucosylceramides and Digalactosyl Diglycerides: A Human Clinical Study." *Cosmetics* 4, no. 4 (September 2017): 37–54. https://www.mdpi.com/2079-9284/4/4/37.

Borumand, Maryam, and Sara Sibilla. "Daily Consumption of the Collagen Supplement Pure Gold Collagen® Reduces Visible Signs of Aging." *Clinical Interventions in Aging* 9 (2014): 1747–58. Dove Medical Press, October 13, 2014. https://www.ncbi.nlm.nih.gov/pmc/articles/PMC4206255.

Boudko, Sergei, Jürgen Engel, Kenji Okuyama, Kazunori Mizuno, and Hans Bächinger. "Crystal Structure of Human Type III Collagen Gly^{991}–Gly^{1032} Cystine Knot-containing Peptide Shows Both 7/2 and 10/3 Triple Helical Symmetries." *Journal of Biological Chemistry* 283 (November 21, 2008): 32580–89. http://www.jbc.org/content/283/47/32580.full.

Buford, Thomas W., Richard B. Kreider, Jeffrey R. Stout, Mike Greenwood, Bill Campbell, Marie Spano, Tim Ziegenfuss, Hector Lopez, Jamie Landis, and Jose Antonio. "International Society of Sports Nutrition Position Stand: Creatine Supplementation and Exercise." *Journal of the International Society of Sports Nutrition* 4, no. 6 (August 30, 2007). https://www.ncbi.nlm.nih.gov/pmc/articles/PMC2048496.

Chua, Lee S., Sze Y. Lee, Norhanisah Abdullah, and Mohamad R. Sarmidi. "Review on Labisia Pumila (Kacip Fatimah): Bioactive Phytochemicals and Skin Collagen Synthesis Promoting Herb." *Fitoterapia* 83, no. 8 (December 2012): 1322–35. https://www.sciencedirect.com/science/article/abs/pii/S0367326X12000949.

Chen, Peiwen, Matilde Cescon, and Paolo Bonaldo. "Lack of Collagen VI Promotes Wound-Induced Hair Growth." *Journal of Investigative Dermatology* 135, no. 10 (June 18, 2015): 2358–67. https://linkinghub.elsevier.com/retrieve/pii/S0022202X15417993.

Chen, Ying, and John Lyga. "Brain-Skin Connection: Stress, Inflammation and Skin Aging." *Inflammation & Allergy Drug Targets* 13, no. 3 (June 2014): 177–90. https://www.ncbi.nlm.nih.gov/pmc/articles/PMC4082169.

Ciccone, Marco Matteo, Francesca Cortese, Michele Gesualdo, Santa Carbonara, Annapaola Zito, Gabriella Ricci, Francesca De Pascalis, Pietro Scicchitano, and Graziano Riccioni. "Dietary Intake of Carotenoids and Their Antioxidant and Anti-Inflammatory Effects in Cardiovascular Care." *Mediators of Inflammation* (2013): 782137. https://www.ncbi.nlm.nih.gov/pmc/articles/PMC3893834.

Clark, Kristine L., Wayne Sebastianelli, Klaus R. Flechsenhar, Douglas F. Aukermann, Felix Meza, Roberta L. Millard, John R. Deitch, Paul S. Sherbondy, and Ann Albert. "24-Week Study on the Use of Collagen Hydrolysate as a Dietary Supplement in Athletes with Activity-Related Joint Pain." *Current Medical Research and Opinion* 24, no. 5 (April 15, 2008): 1485–96. https://www.ncbi.nlm.nih.gov/pubmed/18416885.

Clifford, Tom, Matthew Ventress, Dean M. Allerton, Sarah Stansfield, Jonathan C. Y. Tang, William D. Fraser, Barbara Vanhoecke, Janne Prawitt, and Emma Stevenson. "The Effects of Collagen Peptides on Muscle Damage, Inflammation and Bone Turnover Following Exercise: A Randomized, Controlled Trial." *Amino Acids* 51, no. 4 (February 19, 2019): 691–704. https://www.ncbi.nlm.nih.gov/pubmed/30783776.

Crowley, David C., Francis C. Lau, Prachi Sharma, Malkanthi Evans, Najla Guthrie, Manashi Bagchi, Debasis Bagchi, Dipak K. Dey, and Siba P. Raychaudhuri. "Safety and Efficacy of Undenatured Type II Collagen in the Treatment of Osteoarthritis of the Knee: a Clinical Trial." *International Journal of Medical Sciences* 6, no. 6 (October 9, 2009): 312–21. https://www.ncbi.nlm.nih.gov/pmc/articles/PMC2764342.

Derbyshire, Emma J. "Flexitarian Diets and Health: A Review of the Evidence-Based Literature." *Frontiers in Nutrition* 6, no. 3 (January 2017): 55. https://www.ncbi.nlm.nih.gov/pubmed/28111625.

Elam, Marcus L., Sarah A. Johnson, Shirin Hooshmand, Rafaela G. Feresin, Mark E. Payton, Jennifer Gu, and Bahram H. Arjmandi. "A Calcium-Collagen Chelate Dietary Supplement Attenuates Bone Loss in

Postmenopausal Women with Osteopenia: A Randomized Controlled Trial." *Journal of Medicinal Food* 18, no. 3 (October 14, 2014): 324–31. https://www.ncbi.nlm.nih.gov/pubmed/25314004.

Elisângela, P., and G. B. Fanaro. "Collagen Supplementation as a Complementary Therapy for the Prevention and Treatment of Osteoporosis and Osteoarthritis: a Systematic Review." *Revista Brasileira de Geriatria e Gerontologia* 19, no. 1 (January/February 2016). http://www.scielo.br/scielo.php?script=sci_arttext&pid=S1809-98232016000100153.

Ell, Gorgina, and Brian Lockwood. "Collagen Hydrolysate in Joint Health." *Nutraceutical Business & Technology*, March 1, 2008. https://www.thefreelibrary.com/Collagen hydrolysate in joint health.-a0199464801.

Eutamene, Helene, Catherine Beaufrand, Cheryl Harkat, and Vassilia Theodorou. "The Role of Mucoprotectants in the Management of Gastrointestinal Disorders." *Expert Review of Gastroenterology & Hepatology* 12, no. 1 (September 26, 2017): 83–90. https://www.ncbi.nlm.nih.gov/pubmed/28946778.

Fligiel, Suzanne, James Varani, Subhash Datta, Sewon Kang, Gary Fisher, and John Voorhees. "Collagen Degradation in Aged/Photodamaged Skin In Vivo and After Exposure to Matrix Metalloproteinase-1 In Vitro." *Journal of Investigative Dermatology* 120, no. 5 (May 2003): 824–48. https://www.sciencedirect.com/science/article/pii/S0022202X15302402#bb0135.

Gál, Kat. "Nail Abnormalities: Causes, Symptoms, and Pictures." *Medical News Today*. MediLexicon International, August 10, 2018. https://www.medicalnewstoday.com/articles/322735.php.

Ganceviciene, Ruta, Aikaterini I. Liakou, Athanasios Theodoridis, Evgenia Makrantonaki, and Christos C. Zouboulis. "Skin Anti-Aging Strategies." *Dermato-endocrinology* 4, no. 3 (July 1, 2012): 308–19. https://www.ncbi.nlm.nih.gov/pmc/articles/PMC3583892.

Gardi, Concetta, Beatrice Arezzini, Vittoria Fortino, and Mario Comporti. "Effect of Free Iron on Collagen Synthesis, Cell Proliferation and MMP-2 Expression in Rat Hepatic Stellate Cells." *Biochemical Pharmacology* 64, no. 7 (October 1, 2002): 1139–45. https://www.ncbi.nlm.nih.gov/pubmed/12234617.

Ghouzali, Ibtissem, Caroline Lemaitre, Wafa Bahlouli, Saïda Azhar, Christine Bôle-Feysot, Mathieu Meleine, Philippe Ducrotté, Pierre Déchelotte, and Moïse Coëffier. "Targeting Immunoproteasome and Glutamine Supplementation Prevent Intestinal Hyperpermeability." *Biochimica et Biophysica Acta* 1861, no. 1 Part A, (August 17, 2016): 3278–88. https://www.ncbi.nlm.nih.gov/pubmed/27544233.

Gillies, Allison R., and Richard L. Lieber. "Structure and Function of the Skeletal Muscle Extracellular Matrix." *Muscle & Nerve* 44, no. 3 (September 1, 2011): 318–31. https://www.ncbi.nlm.nih.gov/pmc/articles/PMC3177172.

Grabel, Arielle. "Photoaging: What You Need to Know About the Other Kind of Aging." The Skin Cancer Foundation, January 10, 2019. https://www.skincancer.org/healthy-lifestyle/anti-aging/what-is-photoaging.

Graham, M. F., D. E. Drucker, R. F. Diegelmann, and C. O. Elson. "Collagen Synthesis by Human Intestinal Smooth Muscle Cells in Culture." *Gastroenterology* 92, no. 2 (February 1987): 400–405. https://www.ncbi.nlm.nih.gov/pubmed/3792777.

Harmon, Katherine. "Is Cellulite Forever?" *Scientific American*, May 4, 2009. https://www.scientificamerican.com/article/is-cellulite-forever.

Hashim, P., Mohd Ridzwan, M. S. Baker, J. Hashim, and M. Hashim. "Collagen in Food and Beverage Industries." *International Food Research Journal* 22, no. 1 (2015): 1–8. http://www.ifrj.upm.edu.my/22 (01) 2015/(1).

Hexsel, Doris, Vivian Zague, Michael Schunck, Carolina Siega, Fernanda O. Camozzato, and Steffen Oesser. "Oral Supplementation with Specific Bioactive Collagen Peptides Improves Nail Growth and Reduces Symptoms of Brittle Nails." *Journal of Cosmetic Dermatology* 16, no. 4 (August 8, 2017): 520–26. https://www.ncbi.nlm.nih.gov/pubmed/28786550.

Hines, Jennifer. "Beauty Sleep Is Real! How Lack of Sleep Is Ruining Your Skin." Alaska Sleep Clinic, July 18, 2018. https://www.alaskasleep.com/blog/beauty-sleep-is-real.-how-lack-of-sleep-is-ruining-your-skin.

Hochstenbach-Waelen, Margriet S., Margriet A. B., and Klaas R. "Single-Protein Casein and Gelatin Diets Affect Energy Expenditure Similarly but Substrate Balance and Appetite Differently in Adults." *Journal of Nutrition* 39, no. 12 (December 2009): 2285–92. https://academic.oup.com/jn/article/139/12/2285/4670596.

"How does skin work?" InformedHealth.org. (April 11, 2019). https://www.ncbi.nlm.nih.gov/books/NBK279255.

Huber, Alexander, and Stephen F. Badylak. "Chapter 34: Biological Scaffolds for Regenerative Medicine." In *Principles of Regenerative Medicine*, edited by Anthony Atala, Robert Lanza, Robert Nerem, and James A. Thomsen, 623–35. 2nd edition. Pittsburgh, PA: McGowan Institute for Regenerative Medicine. ScienceDirect. Academic Press, December 13, 2010. https://www.sciencedirect.com/science/article/pii/B9780123814227100343?via=ihub.

InSilicoMeds. "Smoking Accelerates Aging." EurekAlert!, January 16, 2019. https://www.eurekalert.org/pub_releases/2019-01/imi-nss011619.php.

Jugdaohsingha, Ravin, Abigail I. E. Watson, Liliana D. Pedroa, and Jonathan J. Powell. "The Decrease in Silicon Concentration of the Connective Tissues with Age in Rats Is a Marker of Connective Tissue Turnover." *Bone* 75 (June 2015): 40–48. https://www.sciencedirect.com/science/article/pii/S8756328215000411.

Kahan, V., M. L. Andersen, J. Tomimori, and S. Tufik. "Stress, Immunity and Skin Collagen Integrity: Evidence from Animal Models and Clinical Conditions." *Brain, Behavior, and Immunity* 23, no. 8 (November 2009): 1089–95. https://www.ncbi.nlm.nih.gov/pubmed/19523511

Kim, Do-Un, Hee-Chul Chung, Jia Choi, Yasuo Sakai, and Boo-Yong Lee. "Oral Intake of Low-Molecular-Weight Collagen Peptide Improves Hydration, Elasticity, and Wrinkling in Human Skin: A Randomized, Double-Blind, Placebo-Controlled Study." *Nutrients* 10, no. 7 (June 26, 2018): E826. https://www.ncbi.nlm.nih.gov/pubmed/29949889.

Kim, Kyung Eun, Daeho Cho, and Hyun Jeong Park. "Air Pollution and Skin Diseases: Adverse Effects of Airborne Particulate Matter on Various Skin Diseases." *Life Sciences* 1, no. 152 (May 1, 2016): 126–34. https://www.ncbi.nlm.nih.gov/pubmed/27018067.

König, Daniel, Steffen Oesser, Stephan Scharla, Denise Zdzieblik, and Albert Gollhofer. "Specific Collagen Peptides Improve Bone Mineral Density and Bone Markers in Postmenopausal Women—A Randomized Controlled Study." *Nutrients* 10, no. 1 (January 2018): 97. https://www.ncbi.nlm.nih.gov/pmc/articles/PMC5793325.

Kreider, Richard B. "Effects of Creatine Supplementation on Performance and Training Adaptations." *Molecular and Cellular Biochemistry* 224, no. 1–2 (February 2003): 89–94. https://www.ncbi.nlm.nih.gov/pubmed/12701815.

Lan, Annaïg, François Blachier, Robert Benamouzig, Martin Beaumont, Christophe Barrat, Desire Coelho, Antonio Lancha, et al. "Mucosal Healing in Inflammatory Bowel Diseases: Is There a Place for Nutritional Supplementation?" *Inflammatory Bowel Diseases* 21, no. 1 (January 2015): 198–207. https://www.ncbi.nlm.nih.gov/pubmed/25208104.

Larsen, Thomas Meinert, Stine-Mathilde Dalskov, Marleen van Baak, Susan A. Jebb, Angeliki Papadaki, Andreas F. H. Pfeiffer, J. Alfredo Martinez, et al. "Diets with High or Low Protein Content and Glycemic Index for Weight-Loss Maintenance." *New England Journal of Medicine* 363, no. 22 (November 25, 2010): 2102–13. https://www.ncbi.nlm.nih.gov/pubmed/21105792.

Lee, Jin-ah, and Yunhi Cho. "Effect of Ascorbic Acid, Silicon and Iron on Collagen Synthesis in the Human Dermal Fibroblast Cell(HS27)." *FASEB Journal* 22, no. 2, supplement (April 2008). https://www.fasebj.org/doi/abs/10.1096/fasebj.22.2_supplement.672.

Lin, Pei-Hui, Matthew Sermersheim, Haichang Li, Peter H. U. Lee, Steven M. Steinberg, and Jianjie Ma. "Zinc in Wound Healing Modulation." *Nutrients* 10, no. 1 (January 2018): 2–16. https://www.ncbi.nlm.nih.gov/pmc/articles/PMC5793244.

Lin, Meng, Bolin Zhang, Changning Yu, Jiaolong Li, Lin Zhang, Hui Sun, Feng Gao, and Guanghong Zhou. "L-Glutamate Supplementation Improves Small Intestinal Architecture and Enhances the Expressions of Jejunal Mucosa Amino Acid Receptors and Transporters in Weaning Piglets."

PLoS One 9, no. 11 (November 4, 2014): e111950. https://www.ncbi.nlm.nih.gov/pubmed/25368996.

Liu, Xiaoqian, Gustavo C. Machado, Jillian P. Eyles, Varshini Ravi, and David J. Hunter. "Dietary Supplements for Treating Osteoarthritis: A Systematic Review and Meta-Analysis." *British Journal of Sports Medicine* 52, no. 3 (October 10, 2017): 167–75. https://www.ncbi.nlm.nih.gov/pubmed/29018060.

Liu, X., H. Wu, M. Byrne, S. Krane, and R. Jaenisch. "Type III Collagen Is Crucial for Collagen I Fibrillogenesis and for Normal Cardiovascular Development." *Proceedings of the National Academy of Sciences of the United States of America* 94, no. 5 (March 4, 1997): 1852–56. https://www.ncbi.nlm.nih.gov/pmc/articles/PMC20006.

Leonard, Jane. "The Effects of Pollution on Skin." *Aesthetics*, April 6, 2016. https://aestheticsjournal.com/feature/the-effects-of-pollution-on-skin.

Lodish, Harvey, Arnold Berk, S. Lawrence Zipursky, Paul Matsudaira, David Baltimore, and James Darnell. "Collagen: The Fibrous Proteins of the Matrix." In *Molecular Cell Biology*. 4th edition. New York: W. H. Freeman, 2000. https://www.ncbi.nlm.nih.gov/books/NBK21582.

Lopetuso, L. R., F. Scaldaferri, G. Bruno, V. Petito, F. Franceschi, and A. Gasbarrini. "The Therapeutic Management of Gut Barrier Leaking: The Emerging Role for Mucosal Barrier Protectors." *European Review for Medical and Pharmacological Sciences* 19, no. 6 (2015): 1068–1076. https://www.ncbi.nlm.nih.gov/pubmed/25855934.

Lopez, Hector L., Tim N. Ziegenfuss, and Joosang Park. "Evaluation of the Effects of BioCell Collagen, a Novel Cartilage Extract, on Connective Tissue Support and Functional Recovery from Exercise." *Integrative Medicine (Encinitas)* 14, no. 3 (June

2015): 30–38. https://www.ncbi.nlm.nih.gov/pubmed/26770145.

Mast, B. A., R. F. Diegelmann, T. M. Krummel, and I. K. Cohen. "Hyaluronic Acid Modulates Proliferation, Collagen and Protein Synthesis of Cultured Fetal Fibroblasts." *Matrix* 13, no. 6 (November 1993): 441–46. https://www.ncbi.nlm.nih.gov/pubmed/8309423.

MayoClinic. "Placenta: How It Works, What's Normal." Mayo Foundation for Medical Education and Research, April 26, 2018. https://www.mayoclinic.org/healthy-lifestyle/pregnancy-week-by-week/in-depth/placenta/art-20044425.

McEvoy, Claire T., Norman Temple, and Jayne V. Woodside. "Vegetarian Diets, Low-Meat Diets and Health: A Review." *Public Health Nutrition* 15, no. 12 (December 2012): 2287–94. https://www.ncbi.nlm.nih.gov/pubmed/22717188.

McIntosh, James. "Collagen: What Is It and What Are Its Uses?" *Medical News Today.* MediLexicon International, June 16, 2017. https://www.medicalnewstoday.com/articles/262881.php.

Meinke, Martina C., Ceylan K. Nowbary, Sabine Schanzer, Henning Vollert, Jürgen Lademann, and Maxim E. Darvin. "Influences of Orally Taken Carotenoid-Rich Curly Kale Extract on Collagen I/Elastin Index of the Skin." *Nutrients* 9, no. 7 (July 19, 2017): article 775. https://www.ncbi.nlm.nih.gov/pmc/articles/PMC5537889.

Michels, Alexander J. "Vitamin C and Skin Health." Linus Pauling Institute, 2011. https://lpi.oregonstate.edu/mic/health-disease/skin-health/vitamin-C.

Mohammad, Abdul W, Norhazwani M. Suhimi, Abdul Ghani Kumar Abdul Azi, and Jamaliah M. Jahim. "Process for Production of Hydrolysed Collagen from Agriculture Resources: Potential for Further Development."

Journal of Applied Sciences 12, no. 4 (2014): 1319–23. https://scialert.net/fulltextmobile/?doi=jas.2014.1319.1323.

Moskowitz, R. W. "Role of Collagen Hydrolysate in Bone and Joint Disease." *Seminars in Arthritis and Rheumatism* 30, no. 2 (October 2000): 87–99. https://www.ncbi.nlm.nih.gov/pubmed/11071580.

Mukherjee, Siddharth, Abhijit Date, Vandana Patravale, Hans Christian Korting, Alexander Roeder, and Günther Weindl. "Retinoids in the Treatment of Skin Aging: An Overview of Clinical Efficacy and Safety." *Clinical Interventions in Aging* 1, no. 4 (December 2006): 327–48. https://www.ncbi.nlm.nih.gov/pmc/articles/PMC2699641.

National Institutes of Health, U.S. Department of Health and Human Services. "Bone Mass Measurement: What the Numbers Mean." Accessed August 10, 2019. https://www.bones.nih.gov/health-info/bone/bone-health/bone-mass-measure.

Nicita-Mauro, Vittorio, Giorgio Basile, Giuseppe Maltese, Claudio Nicita-Mauro, Sebastiano Gangemi, and Calogero Caruso. "Smoking, Health and Ageing." *Immunity & Aging* 5 (September 16, 2008): 10. https://www.ncbi.nlm.nih.gov/pmc/articles/PMC2564903.

Ohara, Hiroki, Kyoko Ito, Hiroyuki Iida, and Hitoshi Matsumoto. "Improving Skin Stratum Corneum Water Content by Oral Intake of Collagen Peptide." *J-STAGE* 56, no. 3 (2009): 137–45. https://doi.org/10.3136/nskkk.56.137.

Papakonstantinou, Eleni, Michael Roth, and George Karakiulakis. "Hyaluronic Acid: A Key Molecule in Skin Aging." *Dermato-endocrinology* 4, no. 3 (July 1, 2012): 253–58. https://www.ncbi.nlm.nih.gov/pmc/articles/PMC3583886.

Paul, Cristiana, Suzane Leser, and Steffen Oesser. "Significant Amounts of Functional Collagen Peptides Can Be Incorporated in the Diet While Maintaining Indispensable Amino Acid Balance." *Nutrients* 11, no. 5 (May 15, 2019): E1079. https://www.ncbi.nlm.nih.gov/pubmed/31096622.

Pittaoulis, Ann, and Evelyn Phillips. "Can Oral Supplementation with a Collagen-Casein-Based Liquid Protein Improve Serum Albumin Levels in Hemodialysis Patients?" Wiley Online Library. *Dialysis & Transplantation*, April 24, 2007. https://onlinelibrary.wiley.com/doi/full/10.1002/dat.20127.

Posthauer, Mary Ellen. "Conditionally Essential Amino Acids and Nutritional Supplements in Wound Care." WoundSource, December 1, 2017. https://www.woundsource.com/blog/conditionally-essential-amino-acids-and-nutritional-supplements-wound-care.

Proksch, E., D. Segger, J. Degwert, M. Schunck, V. Zague, and S. Oesser. "Oral Supplementation of Specific Collagen Peptides Has Beneficial Effects on Human Skin Physiology: A Double-Blind, Placebo-Controlled Study." *Skin Pharmacology and Physiology* 27 (2014): 47–55. Karger Publishers, August 14, 2013. https://www.karger.com/Article/Abstract/351376.

Proksch, E., M. Schunck, V. Zague, D. Segger, J. Degwert, and S. Oesser. "Oral Intake of Specific Bioactive Collagen Peptides Reduces Skin Wrinkles and Increases Dermal Matrix Synthesis." *Skin Pharmacology and Physiology* 27, no. 3 (December 24, 2014): 113–19. https://www.ncbi.nlm.nih.gov/pubmed/24401291.

Pullar, Juliet M., Anitra C. Carr, and Margreet C. M. Vissers. "The Roles of Vitamin C in Skin Health." *Nutrients* 9, no. 8 (August 12, 2017): 866. https://www.ncbi.nlm.nih.gov/pmc/articles/PMC5579659/pdf/nutrients-09-00866.pdf.

Pugh, Jamie N., Stephen Sage, Mark Hutson, Dominic A. Doran, Simon C. Fleming, Jamie Highton, James P. Morton, and Graeme L. Close. "Glutamine Supplementation Reduces Markers of Intestinal Permeability during Running in the Heat in a Dose-Dependent Manner." *European Journal of Applied Physiology* 117, no. 12 (December 2017): 2569–77. https://www.ncbi.nlm.nih.gov/pubmed/29058112.

Rapin, Jean Robert, and Nicolas Wiernsperger. "Possible Links between Intestinal Permeability and Food Processing: A Potential Therapeutic Niche for Glutamine." *Clinics (Sao Paulo)* 65, no. 6 (June 2010): 635–43. https://www.ncbi.nlm.nih.gov/pmc/articles/PMC2898551.

Rawlings, A. V. "Cellulite and Its Treatment." Wiley Online Library. *International Journal of Cosmetic Science*, May 22, 2006. https://onlinelibrary.wiley.com/doi/full/10.1111/j.1467-2494.2006.00318.x.

Razak, Meerza Abdul, Pathan Shajahan Begum, Buddolla Viswanath, and Senthilkumar Rajagopal. "Multifarious Beneficial Effect of Nonessential Amino Acid, Glycine: A Review." *Oxidative Medicine and Cellular Longevity* (2017): 1716701. https://www.ncbi.nlm.nih.gov/pmc/articles/PMC5350494.

Reeds, Peter J. "Dispensable and Indispensable Amino Acids for Humans." OUP Academic. *Journal of Nutrition* 130, no. 7 (July 1, 2000): 1835S–40S. https://academic.oup.com/jn/article/130/7/1835S/4686195.

Ricard-Blum, Sylvie. "The Collagen Family." *Cold Spring Harbor Perspectives in Biology* 3, no. 1 (January 1, 2011): a004978. https://www.ncbi.nlm.nih.gov/pmc/articles/PMC3003457.

Rubio, I. G., G. Castro, A. C. Zanini, and G. Medeiros-Neto. "Oral Ingestion of a Hydrolyzed Gelatin Meal in Subjects with Normal Weight and in Obese Patients: Postprandial

Effect on Circulating Gut Peptides, Glucose and Insulin." *Eating and Weight Disorders* 13, no. 1 (March 2008): 48–53. https://www.ncbi.nlm.nih.gov/pubmed/18319637.

Samonina, G., L. Lyapina, G. Kopylova, V. Pastorova, Z. Bakaeva, N. Jeliaznik, S. Zuykova, and I. Ashmarin. "Protection of Gastric Mucosal Integrity by Gelatin and Simple Proline-Containing Peptides." *Pathophysiology* 7, no. 1 (April 2000): 69–73. https://www.ncbi.nlm.nih.gov/pubmed/10825688.

Santa Cruz, Jamie. "Dietary Collagen — Should Consumers Believe the Hype?" *Today's Dietitian*, March 2019. https://www.todaysdietitian.com/newarchives/0319p26.shtml.

Scala, J., N. Hollies, and K. Sucher. "Effect of Daily Gelatin Ingestion on Human Scalp Hair." *Nutrition Reports International* 13, no. 6 (January 1976): 579–92. https://www.researchgate.net/publication/279548216_Effect_of_daily_gelatin_ingestion_on_human_scalp_hair.

Schunck, Michael, Vivian Zague, Steffen Oesser, and Ehrhardt Proksch. "Dietary Supplementation with Specific Collagen Peptides Has a Body Mass Index-Dependent Beneficial Effect on Cellulite Morphology." *Journal of Medicinal Food* 18, no. 12 (December 2015): 1340–48. https://www.ncbi.nlm.nih.gov/pubmed/26561784.

Science Learning Hub. "Digestion – Breaking the Large into the Small." Accessed August 2, 2019. https://www.sciencelearn.org.nz/resources/1830-digestion-breaking-the-large-into-the-small.Shaw, Gregory, Ann Lee-Barthel, Megan L. Ross, Bing Wang, and Keith Baar. "Vitamin C-Enriched Gelatin Supplementation before Intermittent Activity Augments Collagen Synthesis." *American Journal of Clinical Nutrition* 105, no. 1 (January 2017): 136–143. https://www.ncbi.nlm.nih.gov/pubmed/27852613.

Shuster, Sam, and Eva McVitie. "The Influence of Age and Sex on Skin Thickness, Skin Collagen and Density." *British Journal of Dermatology* 93, no. 6: (April 1975): 639–43. https://onlinelibrary.wiley.com/doi/pdf/10.1111/j.1365-2133.1975.tb05113.x.

Silva, Tiago H., Joana L. P. Moreira-Silva, Ana L. Marques, Alberta Domingues, Yves Bayon, and Rui L. Reis. "Marine Origin Collagens and Its Potential Applications." *Marine Drugs* 12, no. 12 (December 5, 2014): 5881–901. https://www.ncbi.nlm.nih.gov/pmc/articles/PMC4278207.

Sinclair, Rodney D. "Healthy Hair: What Is It?" *Journal of Investigative Dermatology Symposium Proceedings* 12, no. 2 (December 2007): 2–5. https://www.jidsponline.org/article/S0022-202X(15)52655-9/fulltext.

Söderhäll, Cilla, Ingo Marenholz, Tamara Kerscher, Franz Rüschendorf, Jorge Esparza-Gordillo, Margitta Worm, Christoph Gruber, et al. "Variants in a Novel Epidermal Collagen Gene (COL29A1) Are Associated with Atopic Dermatitis." *PLoS Biology* 5, no. 9 (September 2007): e242. https://www.ncbi.nlm.nih.gov/pmc/articles/PMC1971127.

Soy, Whey, or Whey-GMP." *Clinical Nutrition* 28, no. 2 (April 2009): 147–55. https://www.ncbi.nlm.nih.gov/pubmed/19185957.

Sugihara, Fumihito, Naoki Inoue, and Sriraam Venkateswarathirukumara. "Ingestion of Bioactive Collagen Hydrolysates Enhanced Pressure Ulcer Healing in a Randomized Double-Blind Placebo-Controlled Clinical Study." *Scientific Reports* 8 (2018): 11403. https://www.ncbi.nlm.nih.gov/pmc/articles/PMC6065362.

Tanjore, Harikrishna, and Raghu Kalluri. "The Role of Type IV Collagen and Basement Membranes in Cancer Progression and Metastasis." *American Journal of Pathology* 168, no. 3 (March 2006): 715–17. https://www.ncbi.nlm.nih.gov/pmc/articles/PMC1606530.

Tanoff, Myron, and Joseph Sassani. "Surgical and Nonsurgical Trauma." In *Ocular Pathology*, 93–145. 7th edition. New York: Saunders, 2014. https://www.sciencedirect.com/science/article/pii/B9781455728749000053.

Tariq, M., and A. R. Al Moutaery. "Studies on the Antisecretory, Gastric Anti-Ulcer and Cytoprotective Properties of Glycine." *Research Communications in Molecular Pathology and Pharmacology* 9, no. 2 (August 1997): 185–98. https://www.ncbi.nlm.nih.gov/pubmed/9344231.

Ulrich, P., and A. Cerami. "Protein Glycation, Diabetes, and Aging." *Recent Progress in Hormone Research* 56 (2001): 1–21. https://www.ncbi.nlm.nih.gov/pubmed/11237208.

Varani, James, Michael Dame, Laure Rittie, Suzanne Fligiel, Sewon Kang, Gary Fisher, and John Voorhees. "Decreased Collagen Production in Chronologically Aged Skin: Roles of Age-Dependent Alteration in Fibroblast Function and Defective Mechanical Stimulation." *American Journal of Pathology* 168, no. 6 (June 2006): 1861–68. https://www.ncbi.nlm.nih.gov/pmc/articles/PMC1606623.

Varani, J., R. L. Warner, M. Gharaee-Kermani, S. H. Phan, S. Kang, J. H. Chung, Z. Q. Wang, S. C. Datta, G. J. Fisher, and J. J. Voorhees. "Vitamin A Antagonizes Decreased Cell Growth and Elevated Collagen-Degrading Matrix Metalloproteinases and Stimulates Collagen Accumulation in Naturally Aged Human Skin." *Journal of Investigative Dermatology* 114, no. 3 (March 2000): 480–86. https://www.ncbi.nlm.nih.gov/pubmed/10692106.

Veldhorst, Margriet A. B., Arie G. Nieuwenhuizen, Ananda Hochstenbach-Waelen, Klaas R. Westerterp, Marielle P. K. J. Engelen, Robert-Jan M. Brummer, Nicolaas E. P. Deutz, and Margriet S. Westerterp-Plantenga. "A Breakfast with Alpha-Lactalbumin, Gelatin, or Gelatin TRP Lowers Energy Intake at Lunch Compared with a Breakfast

with Casein, Wong, M., M. J. Hendrix, K. von der Mark, C. Little, and R. Stern. "Collagen in the Egg Shell Membranes of the Hen." *Developmental Biology* (July 1984): 28–36. https://www.ncbi.nlm.nih.gov/pubmed/6203793.

Viguet-Carrin, S., P. Garnero, and P. D. Delmas. "The Role of Collagen in Bone Strength." *Osteoporosis International* 17, no. 3 (2006): 319–36. https://www.ncbi.nlm.nih.gov/pubmed/16341622.

Wang, Bin, Guoyao Wu, Zhigang Zhou, Zhaolai Dai, Yuli Sun, Yun Ji, Wei Li, et al. "Glutamine and Intestinal Barrier Function." *Amino Acids* 47, no. 10 (October 2015): 2143–54. https://www.ncbi.nlm.nih.gov/pubmed/24965526.

Wang, Bin, Zhenlong Wu, Yun Ji, Kaiji Sun, Zhaolai Dai, and Guoyao Wu. "L-Glutamine Enhances Tight Junction Integrity by Activating CaMK Kinase 2-AMP-Activated Protein Kinase Signaling in Intestinal Porcine Epithelial Cells." *Journal of Nutrition* 146, no. 3 (March 2016): 501–8. https://www.ncbi.nlm.nih.gov/pubmed/26865645.

World Health Organization. "Q&A on the Carcinogenicity of the Consumption of Red Meat and Processed Meat." May 17, 2016. https://www.who.int/features/qa/cancer-red-meat/en.

Wu, Guoyao, Fuller W. Bazer, Robert C. Burghardt, Gregory A. Johnson, Sung Woo Kim, Darrell A. Knabe, Peng Li, et al. "Proline and Hydroxyproline Metabolism: Implications for Animal and Human Nutrition." *Amino Acids* 40, no. 4 (April 2011): 1053–63. https://www.ncbi.nlm.nih.gov/pmc/articles/PMC3773366.

Yamauchi, K, Y Matsumoto, and K Yamauchi. "Egg Collagen Content Is Increased by a Diet Supplemented with Wood Charcoal Powder Containing Wood Vinegar Liquid." *British Poultry Science* 57, no. 5 (October

2016): 601–11. https://www.ncbi.nlm.nih.gov/pubmed/27376436.

Yamamoto, T., N. Iwashila, K. Maeda, E. Nishimura, K. Notake, N. Naoi, and S. Yano. "Effects of Oral Intake of Porcine Skin Collagen Peptides on Moisture and Robustness of Fingernail—A Randomized, Double-blind, Placebo-controlled Study." *Japanese Pharmacology and Therapeutics* 45, no. 11 (January 2017): 1787–93. https://www.researchgate.net/publication/322198845.

Yang, F. C., Y. C. Zhang, and M. Rheinstädter. "The Structure of People's Hair." *PeerJ* 2 (October 14, 2014): e619. https://www.ncbi.nlm.nih.gov/pmc/articles/PMC4201279.

Yoon, Hyun-Sun, Hyun Cho, Se-Rah Lee, Mi-Hee Shin, and Jin Chung. "Supplementating with Dietary Astaxanthin Combined with Collagen Hydrolysate Improves Facial Elasticity and Decreases Matrix Metalloproteinase-1 and -12 Expression: A Comparative Study with Placebo." *Journal of Medicinal Food* 17, no. 7 (June 23, 2014): 810–16. https://www.ncbi.nlm.nih.gov/pubmed/24955642.

Zdzieblik, Denise, Steffen Oesser, Manfred W. Baumstark, Albert Gollhofer, and Daniel König. "Collagen Peptide Supplementation in Combination with Resistance Training Improves Body Composition and Increases Muscle Strength in Elderly Sarcopenic Men: A Randomised Controlled Trial." British Journal of Nutrition 114, no. 8 (October 28, 2015): 1237–45. https://www.ncbi.nlm.nih.gov/pmc/articles/PMC4594048.

Index

ABOUT THE AUTHOR

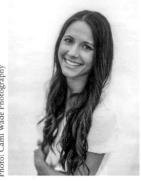

Jessica Bippen, MS, RD, is a registered dietitian who believes in a whole-person approach to wellness and balanced living. She is the founder of Nourished by Nutrition, a wellness website where she shares delicious, healthy recipes and science-based nutrition information. Her mission is to help women uncover their forever wellness for every season of life. Bippen is a nutrition expert at HUM nutrition and for the Tammy Hembrow Fitness app. Her work has been featured on the HUM blog, Free People, and Well + Good, among others. Visit Jessica at nourishedbynutrition.com.